Clinical Cases in Dermatology

For further volumes:
http://www.springer.com/series/10473

Robert A. Norman • Reena Rupani

Clinical Cases in Integrative Dermatology

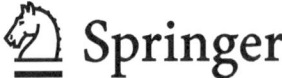 Springer

Robert A. Norman
Dermatology Healthcare
Tampa, FL
USA

Reena Rupani
Department of Dermatology
SUNY Downstate Medical
Center
Brooklyn, NY
USA

ISBN 978-3-319-10243-6   ISBN 978-3-319-10244-3   (eBook)
DOI 10.1007/978-3-319-10244-3
Springer Cham Heidelberg New York Dordrecht London

Library of Congress Control Number: 2014952791

Printed on acid-free paper

Springer is part of Springer Science+Business Media (www.springer.com)

Preface

We are happy and privileged to present dermatology clinical cases in the cutting edge field of integrative dermatology. If you are new to the field, you will begin to develop a literacy and competence in integrative dermatology. By becoming familiar with more healing systems beyond medical dermatology, you can put additional modalities into your therapeutic tool chest. For the more experienced learner, you will hopefully find new ways to sharpen your diagnostic and treatment acumen.

Integrative dermatology therapies have steadily increased in popularity and a significant percentage of the population has incorporated integrative dermatology into daily use. We hope that each chapter can serve as a springboard for further pursuit and more extensive training.

I was honored to help start the curriculum in integrative dermatology at the Arizona Center for Integrative Medicine at the University of Arizona College of Medicine founded by Dr. Andrew Weil where Dr. Rupani completed her fellowship. Whenever possible we lecture and mentor students in our local medical schools and our offices on the wonders of integrative dermatology. We hope that this book and others to follow will help bring the knowledge of integrative dermatology to a wider audience.

Inside the covers of this book you will find very useful information and tools to help your patients, adding to your current clinical regimen with everything from breath work, meditation and yoga to barberry root. We hope this text provides help and insight for you and your patients in handling the skin and its contents.

– Rob Norman

As Thomas Edison once famously said:

"The doctor of the future will give no medicine, but will instruct his patient in the care of the human frame, in diet and in the cause and prevention of disease."

Those of us who are trained in Western allopathic medicine may find it difficult or unnatural to "give no medicine"—as such, the field of integrative medicine, which combines all approaches to healing and attempts to act under evidence-based guidance, is a holistic approach to patient care.

Integrative dermatology is a relatively newly-defined field, but one for which many of our patients clamor: our acne patients often seek dietary counseling, our photo-damaged patients ask about botanical extracts and cosmeceuticals, our patients struggling with hyperhidrosis wonder "what else" they can try.

This clinical case book was therefore compiled to hopefully serve as a useful guide for dermatologists, internists, family practitioners, pediatricians, and anyone else charged with the care of the skin. The case-based format aims to distinguish this work from a reference-style textbook, and instead allow readers to identify something of their own patients in these pages.

I hope this book finds a happy home in your lab coat pocket, or on your medical bookshelf.

Tampa, FL, USA   Rob Norman
Brooklyn, NY, USA   Reena Rupani

Contents

Authors and Contributors

Authors

Robert A. Norman   Dermatology Healthcare, Tampa, FL, USA

Reena Rupani   Department of Dermatology, SUNY Downstate Medical Center, Brooklyn, NY, USA

Contributors

Patrick Brennan   Lake Erie College of Osteopathic Medicine, Bradenton, FL, USA

Jaime B. Glick   Department of Dermatology, SUNY Downstate Medical Center, Brooklyn, NY, USA

Laura Jordan   Lake Erie College of Osteopathic Medicine, Bradenton, FL, USA

Raman Madan   Department of Dermatology, SUNY Downstate Medical Center, Brooklyn, NY, USA

Chapter 1
A 16 Year Old with Hair Loss

Reena Rupani

A 16-year-old girl presents to a pediatrician with significant distress surrounding acute hair loss. She says for the past few weeks she has been losing "clumps" of hair on her pillow, in her shower, and in her hair brush. She typically washes her hair every day, but recently has decreased to once weekly out of a desire to mitigate the loss. She is only combing with a wide-toothed comb, and does not use any styling products. She is very anxious and upset about her loss of hair. She is accompanied by her mother and two younger sisters.

Her past medical history is significant for rheumatic fever as a child, but she does not take any medications or supplements regularly. There is no family history of hair loss. She is the eldest of five siblings, and describes her family as "involved" and Catholic. She is in the 11th grade and is a good student, planning to attend college and pursue studies in literature after she graduates. She eats most of her meals at home (except for school lunches), and has several close friends. Her mother describes her as "bookish."

On physical exam, the patient is appropriately developed for her age, and visibly anxious. A hair pull test reveals five

R. Rupani
Department of Dermatology, SUNY Downstate Medical Center,
Brooklyn, NY, USA
e-mail: reena_rupani@yahoo.com

R.A. Norman, R. Rupani, *Clinical Cases in Integrative Dermatology*, Clinical Cases in Dermatology 4, DOI 10.1007/978-3-319-10244-3_1, © Springer International Publishing Switzerland 2015

and then six hairs on sequential trials. She states that she last washed her hair yesterday. There is some thinning noted over the bitemporal regions of the scalp, but otherwise her hair is relatively thick and dense. There are no areas of frank alopecia, and no scarring is noted on the scalp. Her review of systems is otherwise fully negative.

Differential Diagnosis

1. Lupus
2. Trichotillomania
3. Telogen effluvium
4. Androgenetic alopecia

Lupus: In systemic lupus, hair loss/thinning is often described by patients. Serum ANA is typically positive, and by review of systems or laboratory analysis, the patient should also meet other criteria for lupus. A scalp biopsy may help confirm the diagnosis if clinically suspicious.

Trichotillomania: This condition is defined by patients (either consciously or not) pulling out their own hair, often in conjunction with anxiety or depression. In a more subtle version of this condition, patients may pull or twist their hair habitually, gradually leading to loss. Patterns of hair loss are typically more focal.

Telogen effluvium: The hair growth cycle consists of three phases: anagen (active growth), catagen (transition/resting), and telogen (shedding). Following severe stress, illness, hospitalization, surgery, or pregnancy, patients may notice dramatic shedding of telogen hairs. This typically occurs approximately 3 months after the inciting event. Laboratory workup should be within normal limits, and while this is typically a clinical diagnosis, a scalp biopsy may reveal greater proportions of telogen hairs. A hair pull test should be performed on a day when the patient has not shampooed, and a positive result would be the extraction of 6 or more hairs out of a group of 40 hairs pulled. While typically a self-limiting

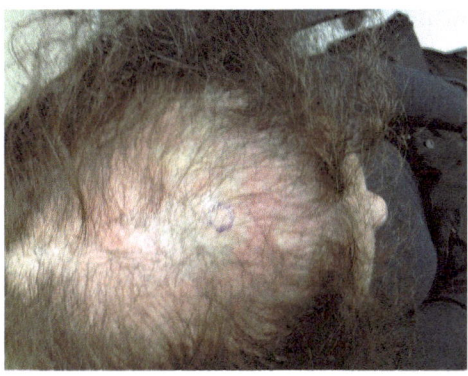

FIGURE 1.1 Diffuse hair loss as can been seen in advanced telogen effluvium

problem (with resolution of normal hair thickness and growth within 3–6 months), some cases of telogen effluvium can become chronic and unmask an underlying tendency towards androgenetic alopecia (Fig. 1.1).

Androgenetic alopecia: Commonly referred to as "male pattern baldness," androgenetic alopecia can occur in female patients as well, and can be seen in younger age groups. Male pattern is typically more over the bitemporal region and vertex, whereas female pattern preserves the anterior hairline and begins as widening of the part, progressing to diffuse thinning over the top of the scalp. Thyroid function, iron status, and vitamin D levels should be assessed and optimized. The etiology of androgenetic alopecia is thought to be multifactorial, with components of genetics, hormone levels, and environmental factors playing a role. Onset is usually insidious and progressive.

Further Workup The patient's family is asked to return to the waiting room, so that the doctor can perform a private examination. Her mother is initially resistant but later acquiesces. The pediatrician then takes the opportunity to spend a few more minutes on the patient's history, and asks if anything particularly stressful has occurred in the last several months. The patient denies anything out of the ordinary. Her doctor then asks if she is sexually active, and the patient breaks down in tears. She admits to having a boyfriend of which her parents are not aware, as they are quite controlling and resistant to dating, and states that she had protected sexual intercourse for the first (and only) time 3 months ago. She has been feeling incredibly guilty and anxious since that event, to the point that her boyfriend broke up with her last week.

A serum vitamin D level, CBC, iron studies, and TSH are all found to be within normal limits. Beta-HcG and ANA are negative.

Diagnosis   Telogen effluvium

Conventional Treatment Options

- **Time**: The natural course of telogen effluvium is resolution, typically within 3–6 months, although some cases can become chronic (particularly if the patient has underlying androgenetic alopecia which becomes unmasked). Most often, however, if the inciting factor was an isolated event or occurrence, then full resolution without intervention is typical.
- **Counseling**: If telogen effluvium is secondary to (or accompanied by) severe stress or anxiety, referral for professional counseling may help break the vicious cycle.
- **Minoxidil**: Topical minoxidil is available in 2 and 5 % formulations, and while the approved indication is for androgenetic alopecia, may help promote hair growth in telogen effluvium as well (use is off-label). One caution with minoxidil is that, for androgenetic alopecia, cessation of treatment leads to shedding of any regained hairs—this phenomenon, however, is not clear-cut in acute telogen effluvium but remains a possibility of which patients should be aware. Additionally, minoxidil is available in

solution and foam formulations, and many patients report irritation with the former (likely from the propylene glycol in the vehicle).

Integrative Treatment Options

- **Avoidance of products containing parabens, sulphates, and phthalates**: To generally support healthy hair and discourage breakage of newly growing strands, it is advisable to use hair care products that are as free of potential irritants and carcinogenic or endocrine-disrupting chemicals as possible.
- **Eucalyptus oil**: The benefits of eucalyptus oil are more in supporting the elasticity and shine of existing hair, rather than promoting new hair growth [1], but this effect in turn can improve the patient's perception of their hair and reduce the surrounding anxiety of telogen effluvium. Eucalyptus is presently available in commercial "root awakening" formulas.
- **Coconut oil**: Contrary to some cultural beliefs, coconut oil does not demonstrate the ability to grow new hair, but rather supports the health of that which is already existing. This oil has the highest ability to penetrate inside the hair shaft based on low molecular weight and linear structure, thus preventing protein loss and improving hair strength and appearance [2].
- **Breathwork**: Several forms of breathwork, developed and taught by the Arizona Center for Integrative Medicine [3], can serve to allay the anxiety that often accompanies chronic pruritus and feeds into a vicious cycle. The overall goal is to slow down and deepen the breath.

  - 4-7-8 breath: Patients are counseled to breathe in for a count of 4, hold the breath for a count of 7, then breathe out for a count of 8. The ratios matter more than the speed of the breath, and this should be repeated for four cycles, twice daily.

- – Square breathing: Patients are instructed to imagine that over two breath cycles (in, out, in, out) they are drawing the four sides of a square.
- – "I am, at peace": With each inhale, the patient thinks, "I am," and with each exhale, "at peace."

- **Ashwagandha**: *Withania somnifera* is among the family of "adaptogens," or herbs that help to bidirectionally normalize metabolic and endocrine functions to reduce stress and return the body to homeostasis [4]. Ashwagandha has been used as an anxiolytic and stress reducer for adults and children in Ayurvedic medicine for thousands of years, and dosing is standardized to the percentage of active withanolides. Its use is inadvisable during pregnancy or breastfeeding, and in large doses it can cause gastrointestinal side effects. Additionally, it is not known whether ashwagandha could increase the activity of the immune system in autoimmune disease states such as lupus or rheumatoid arthritis. Thirdly, ashwagandha should be stopped 2 weeks prior to scheduled surgery, as it could potentiate the effects of general anesthesia [5].
- **Ginseng**: Another adaptogen, *Panax ginseng* has also demonstrated the ability to grow hair [6, 7]. So far only one human clinical trial has been published but it showed that oral consumption of Korean red ginseng extract (3,000 mg/day) for 24 weeks effectively increased hair density and thickness in alopecia patients [8].
- **Biotin**: A common ingredient in supplements purported to promote hair strength and growth, biotin is used anecdotally in doses ranging from 1 to 5 mg daily among patients with various forms of hair loss. True biotin deficiency in the absence of congenital enzymatic disorders is rare, and the evidence for its use in otherwise healthy patients with alopecia is weak [9]. Still, many patients choose to take biotin supplements, as it confers a positive sense of agency in their disease, with low risk of toxicity.

Discussion

The patient was reassured that her hair loss is temporary and most likely to resolve within the next few months. It was explained to her mother that, while the medical workup was all normal, the patient has been dealing with significant emotional stress which is manifesting as hair loss. The details of this stress were not shared at the time, but the family was referred to a psychologist, with the idea that family counseling might improve levels of communication and understanding at home.

Additionally, she was advised to look for hair care products that are all-natural and free of chemical additives. She was interested in taking biotin supplements (1,000 mcg daily starting dose), and also planned to perform twice weekly deep conditioning treatments with coconut oil to support hair strength.

Finally, she agreed to reserve some daily time for herself, and was taught the 4-7-8 breath.

References

1. Mamada A, Ishihama M, Fukuda R, Inoue S. Changes in hair properties by Eucalyptus extract. J Cosmet Sci. 2008;59:481–96.
2. Rele AS, Mohile RB. Effect of mineral oil, sunflower oil, and coconut oil on prevention of hair damage. J Cosmet Sci. 2003;54:175–92.
3. Weil, Andrew. The benefits of breathwork. Retrieved on 27 Jan 2014 from www.azcim.org
4. Winston D, Maimes S. Adaptogens: herbs for strength, stamina, and stress relief. Vermont: Inner Traditions/Bear & Co; 2007.
5. Ashwagandha: Uses, side effects, interactions, and warnings. Retrieved on 27 Jan 2014 from www.webMD.com
6. Matsuda H, Yamazaki M, Asanuma Y, Kubo M. Promotion of hair growth by Ginsenz Radix on cultured mouse vibrissal hair follicles. Phytother Res. 2003;17:797–800.
7. Park S, Shin W-S, Ho J. Fructus panax ginseng extract promotes hair regeneration in C57BL/6 mice. J Ethnopharm. 2011;138:340–4.

8. Kim JH, Yi SM, Choi JE, Son SW. Study of the efficacy of Korean red ginseng in the treatment of androgenic alopecia. J Ginseng Res. 2009;33:223–8.
9. Goldberg LJ, Lenzy Y. Nutrition and hair. Clin Dermatol. 2010;28(4):412–9.

Chapter 2
33 Year Old Man
with Growths on His Fingers

Reena Rupani

Case Presentation

A 33-year-old man presents for evaluation of several growths on his fingers in the last year. It began as one lesion and subsequently he has noticed four more. They are occasionally itchy or painful, and have not responded to over-the-counter treatments, including 40 % salicylic acid plaster or "freeze off" therapies. He denies any other medical problems, medications, or drug allergies.

He works in construction, and sometimes finds that the warts get rubbed and irritated by his heavy-duty gloves. He also admits to feeling embarrassed to shake people's hands. He is interested in an "aggressive" treatment but also expresses a curiosity about hypnosis—a neighbor suggested it to him.

On examination, he is an overweight male with diffusely dry skin. His bilateral thumbs and left second digit have five large cauliflower-like verrucous plaques in a periungual distribution, with some noted dystrophy of the adjacent nail plates.

R. Rupani
Department of Dermatology, SUNY Downstate Medical Center,
Brooklyn, NY, USA
e-mail: reena_rupani@yahoo.com

R.A. Norman, R. Rupani, *Clinical Cases in Integrative Dermatology*, Clinical Cases in Dermatology 4, DOI 10.1007/978-3-319-10244-3_2, © Springer International Publishing Switzerland 2015

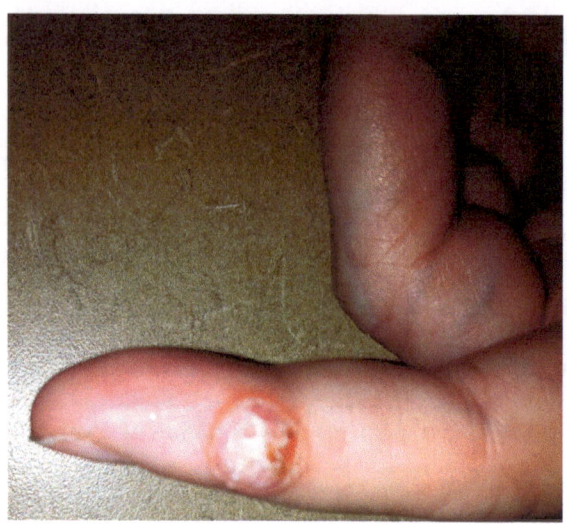

FIGURE 2.1 Verrucous papules on the hands

Diagnosis Verruca vulgaris

Further Workup Not indicated

Discussion

Verruca vulgaris (warts; Fig. 2.1) are benign skin growths caused by human papilloma virus, of which there are more than 100 serotypes. Different strains of the virus tend to have a predilection for different anatomic regions (glabrous versus non-glabrous skin, etc.)—common warts are typically caused by HPV 2 and 4, and genital warts are most attributed to HPV 6, 11, 16, and 18 (the latter two most associated with squamous cell carcinomas of genital and cervical epithelia). Verrucae may be planar, cerebriform, filiform, or cystic in appearance. Diagnosis is typically based on clinical evaluation, but histopathology may be useful in differentiating large/recalcitrant lesions from verrucous carcinoma. In cases of extensive warts, a workup for immunodeficiency or compromise may be indicated.

Conventional treatment options are many, in that none is universally or predictably effective. Use of chemical therapies should be avoided in pregnant or breast-feeding women. A treatment algorithm would be generally as follows:

- Topical salicylic acid solutions, gels, and plasters (ranging from 17 % to 40 %, available over the counter)
- Paring—Using a 15-blade in the office, warts can be pared or shaved to the level of the lower epidermis (visualization of "bleeding points" or dermal capillaries is an endpoint). This allows for better penetration of medication or cryotherapy. At home, patients can be instructed to self-pare using a nail file or dull blade.
- Liquid nitrogen application/cryotherapy—Liquid nitrogen is inexpensive, quick to apply, effective, and cold (−321 °F). Typically it requires several sessions spaced apart by 2–4 weeks for maximum efficacy, and each session may include two to three cycles of application with a 10 s thaw time per cycle.
- Electrocautery—Using an electrodesiccator device, warts can be cauterized and removed. One should ideally take care to use a smoke evacuator system, to minimize both patient and practitioner exposure to aerosolized HPV particles in the generated smoke plume.
- 5-fluorouracil—This topical chemotherapeutic cream has virucidal properties and is available by prescription. It can be combined or alternated with salicylic acid to increase epidermal penetration.
- Imiquimod—Imiquimod (Aldara™) 5 % cream is an immunomodulator that is Food and Drug Administration (FDA) approved for use for genital and perianal warts in patients 12 years or older. It induces skin cells to secrete interferon alpha and other cytokines. It can also be used off-label for non-genital warts, with less reliable efficacy.
- Cantharidin/ podophyllin resin—Office-applied compounds secreted by the blister beetle and American May

Apple tree, respectively, they cause blistering and necrosis of involved skin. Several treatments may be required.

– Podophyllotoxin—This is a cytotoxic compound that tends to work better on mucosal surfaces and is used more commonly in the treatment of genital warts. Patients may apply it topically twice daily for 3 consecutive days per week and repeated weekly, not to exceed 4 weeks.

– Sinecatechins—Veregen™ 15 % ointment is a water extract of green tea leaves from *Camellia sinensis*. It has been shown to inhibit enzymes related to viral replication, and is approved for use on genital warts.

– TCA—Trichloroacetic acid is another means of physical destruction, via chemical coagulation of proteins.

– Intralesional interferon, candida antigen, or bleomycin—The first two are considered forms of intralesional immunotherapy, whereas bleomycin is directly cytotoxic.

– Oral cimetidine—At high doses, this type-2 histamine receptor antagonist displays immunomodulatory properties and may therefore treat warts; however, efficacy is variable. Dosing in adults and children is 20–40 mg/kg orally per day in divided doses every 6 h, not to exceed 2,400 mg/day in adults. There are many known drug interactions with cimetidine, so this medication should be used with caution.

– Photodynamic therapy—Aminolevulinic acid is a photosensitizing chemical that can be used topically in combination with red or blue light, as an off-label treatment for verruca plana or other non-genital warts.

– Shaving—Warts can be physically shaved off with a surgical blade (and specimens sent for pathology confirmation), but the presence of HPV in surrounding skin is often high thereby leading to a significant rate of recurrence. Additionally, scarring is a concern.

– Laser (vascular or ablative)—The most expensive of the conventional treatment options, both vascular and ablative carbon dioxide lasers can be used to treat warts. These procedures are not likely to be covered by insurance and are also not without a rate of recurrence. Again, one should utilize a smoke evacuator during the procedure.

– Biopsy—For warts that are especially large or resistant to therapy, consider a biopsy to rule out verrucous carcinoma.

An integrative approach to treatment would include several other options for non-responders to standard therapy:

– Adhesiotherapy: This refers to the mechanical keratolysis that occurs with the overnight application and removal of heavy adhesive tape, such as the silver-colored mechanical duct tape. Although two randomized controlled trials did not show efficacy over placebo tape [1, 2] other studies have demonstrated a benefit [3]. This method can also be combined with topical keratolytics and cytotoxic agents, such as salicylic acid and fluorouracil cream (see above).
– Hypnosis: Suggestion and its associated placebo effect have a long history of enhancing wart resolution both in folklore and in the medical literature [4, 5]. The concept is that belief can change brain electrochemistry, leading to modification of cell-mediated immunity through psycho-neuro-endocrine effects on the immune system [6].
– Botanical approaches: Raw garlic cloves have been shown to have antiviral activity and can be rubbed onto the wart nightly, followed by occlusion [7]. Topical tea tree oil has also been reported as successful in some cases [8].

Case Discussion The patient was treated with liquid nitrogen cryotherapy in the office after a discussion about risks, which here included permanent nail dystrophy. He was then given a nightly home regimen consisting of the following: (1) Soaking the hands in warm water for 5 min, (2) Using a nail file or dull blade to pare away the dead skin, (3) Applying fluorouracil 5 % cream to the warts under duct tape occlusion at bedtime, alternating nights with over the counter 17 % salicylic acid liquid to the warts under occlusion. He was unable to locate a true medical hypnosis practitioner where he lived, but he was coached to employ mindfulness and positive intention at home, actively envisioning his immune system fighting off the warts each night during the soaking/paring routine. He was seen subsequently for two more sessions of cryotherapy spaced apart by 4 weeks each, and by the fourth office visit, his warts had completely resolved.

References

1. Wenner R, Askari SK, Cham PM, Kedrowski DA, Liu A, Warshaw EM. Duct tape for the treatment of common warts in adults: a double-blind randomized controlled trial. Arch Dermatol. 2007;143(3):309–13.
2. de Haen M, Spigt M, van Uden C, van Neer P, Feron FJ, Knottnerus A. Efficacy of duct tape vs placebo in the treatment of verruca vulgaris (warts) in primary school children. Arch Pediatr Adolesc Med. 2006;160(11):1121–5.
3. Focht 3rd DR, Spicer C, Fairchok MP. The efficacy of duct tape vs cryotherapy in the treatment of verruca vulgaris (the common wart). Arch Pediatr Adolesc Med. 2002;156(10):971–4.
4. Bloch B. Über die heilung der warzen durch suggestion. J Mol Med. 1927;6(49):2320–5.
5. Sulzberger MB, Wolf J. The treatment of warts by suggestion. New York: Medical Record; 1934.
6. Shenefelt PD. Hypnosis in dermatology. Arch Dermatol. 2000;136(3):393.
7. Silverberg NB. Garlic cloves for verruca vulgaris. Pediatr Dermatol. 2002;19(2):183.
8. Millar BC, Moore JE. Successful topical treatment of hand warts in a paediatric patient with tea tree oil (Melaleuca alternifolia). Complement Ther Clin Pract. 2008;14(4):225–7.

Chapter 3
53 Year Old Man
with Chronic Itching

Reena Rupani

A 53-year-old man comes in complaining of a chronic itchy sensation "everywhere on my body." Scratching is the only thing that makes him feel better. He has been struggling with this symptom for the past year, and it has been progressively worsening. He does not notice a seasonal variation.

He is originally from the Ukraine but has been in the United States for the past 10 years, working as a taxi driver. He spends his days driving, which he says makes him feel sweaty and dirty. He typically takes hot showers twice daily for about 30 min at a time, using antibacterial soaps and a washcloth. He does not use a moisturizer as he dislikes the sticky feeling on his skin. His wife does the laundry, and he says she tends to buy whichever detergent and fabric softener are on sale.

The patient is married, has three children, and eats a diet of primarily meat and potatoes. He has not visited a doctor in quite some time and is not up to date on routine health screens such as a prostate exam and colonoscopy, although his review of systems is non-revealing. He denies any medications and is allergic to sulfa. He does not drink alcohol, as his father died of liver cirrhosis, but does smoke one pack per day of cigarettes.

R. Rupani
Department of Dermatology, SUNY Downstate Medical Center,
Brooklyn, NY, USA
e-mail: reena_rupani@yahoo.com

R.A. Norman, R. Rupani, *Clinical Cases in Integrative Dermatology*, Clinical Cases in Dermatology 4,
DOI 10.1007/978-3-319-10244-3_3,
© Springer International Publishing Switzerland 2015

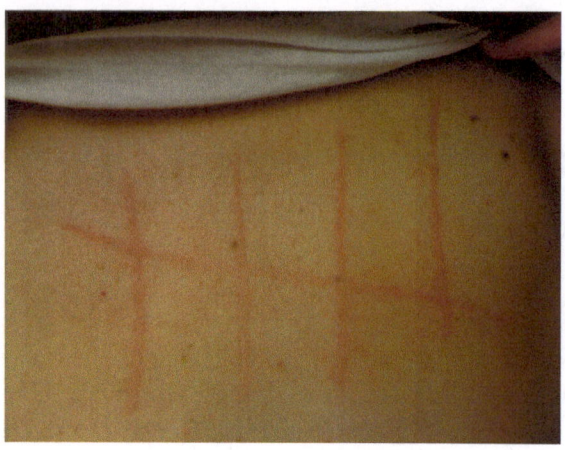

FIGURE 3.1 Dermatographism in the setting of diffuse pruritis

His physical exam reveals moderately dry, flaky skin throughout, and some fissures on his palms. Heavy excoriations are noted, particularly on the legs.

Differential Diagnosis

1. Primary cutaneous pruritus
2. Secondary pruritus
3. Neurodermatitis
4. Allergic contact dermatitis

Primary cutaneous pruritus—Itching that comes directly from a cutaneous origin is termed primary cutaneous pruritus. The most common causative factor is xerosis, often with a component of irritant dermatitis which exacerbates the underlying problem. Patients who are experiencing itch will often try to soothe their symptoms with hot showers and vigorous scrubbing, and use of highly fragranced soaps and detergents can worsen the feeling. Additionally, failing to moisturize the skin properly can be contributory. In some cases, excess circulating histamine can contribute to pruritus, and may be demonstrated by the phenomenon of dermatographism (Fig. 3.1).

Secondary pruritus—Secondary pruritus refers to that which stems from an internal source, such as a metabolic abnormality (hypothyroidism, diabetes, liver or kidney disease), polycythemia, or a paraneoplastic phenomenon in malignancy (specifically non-Hodgkins lymphoma). The review of systems and past medical history are important guides for this diagnosis, as is basic labwork including a complete blood count, metabolic profile, liver function testing, and chest radiography. Age-appropriate malignancy screening such as colonoscopy and mammography should be up to date.

Neurodermatitis—Also known as lichen simplex chronicus, neurodermatitis is a disorder characterized by excessive, vigorous scratching to relieve an itch that can be cutaneous, neuropathic, or psychogenic in origin. The sensation of itch is typically focal/localized, and limited to areas that a patient can reach.

Allergic contact dermatitis—This form of itching is directly attributable to an external causative factor, and tends to have an acute onset. Typically the skin will exhibit signs of inflammation, such as erythema and/or vesiculation.

Further Workup Routine blood work including CBC, chemistry panel, and thyroid function are performed, and found to be normal. A chest x-ray is non-revealing. The patient is referred to a primary care physician for a physical exam, PSA, and colonoscopy which are also non-revealing.

Diagnosis Primary cutaneous pruritus

Conventional Treatment Options

• Gentle skin care—The cornerstone of treatment for itchy skin is to first ensure that patients are properly moisturizing, and also not overly irritating their skin with scented products and harsh cleansing techniques. Mild non-soap cleansers (such as unscented Dove™ or Cetaphil™) are recommended; patients are advised to limit their bath or shower to lukewarm water, and only 5–10 min in duration; patients should use only their hands to apply soap (instead of loofahs or washcloths), and for those with very dry skin, should only apply soap to axillae, groin, and feet; and finally, thick unscented emollients (instead of lotions or oils) should be applied immediately after bathing to wet skin (some examples include Cetaphil™ cream, petroleum jelly, Aquaphor™, Eucerin™, or Aveeno™). Finally, laundry care is part of gentle skin care practices, and recommendations include fragrance-free/dye-free products (such as ALL Free and Clear™ or Seventh Generation™), avoiding fabric softeners, and using only unscented dryer sheets.

- Antihistamines—As histamine is one of the primary mediators of itch, suppressive therapy can be helpful for symptom relief (but is rarely curative). Typical doses would be diphenhydramine 25 mg PO qhs, or hydroxyzine 10–25 mg PO qhs. Caution should be exercised in those who are on other sedating medications, in the elderly, or those with hepatic disease.
- Rule out systemic causes—If the review of systems indicates concern for metabolic or neoplastic phenomena, then appropriate blood work and screening examinations should be performed. Additionally, for patients who return for a follow-up visit and appear to have well-hydrated skin and are following good skin care practices, but are still complaining of pruritus, further workup is warranted.

Integrative Treatment Options

- Burdock-Long used in traditional Chinese medicine, as well as naturopathic medicine, burdock *(Arctium lappa)* is a "blood purifier" that has skin applications. It is known to be rich in phytosterols and long-chain essential fatty acids [1], and also has the ability to limit mast cell degranulation and release of histamine [2]. Burdock should be avoided in pregnant women (as it has some uterine stimulating properties), as well as those with allergies to other members of the Asteraceae family. Safety in children or nursing mothers has not been established, and burdock may interfere with insulin action in diabetics [3, 4]. Burdock can be taken as an oral supplement (although doses are not standardized for primary cutaneous pruritus), and can also be found in several over-the-counter emollients for topical use.

- Calendula: Also known as "pot marigold," *Calendula officinalis* is another member of the Asteraciae family with documented benefits in wound healing [5] and dermatitis [6]. Studies are lacking specifically for pruritus, but its anti-inflammatory triterpinoids [7] anecdotally confer healing to itchy skin. It is available in topical emollient formulations, such as brands including California Baby™ and Weleda™. Potential side effects would include allergic contact dermatitis.

- Aloe: *Aloe barbadensis* is historically known for its role in wound healing and burn treatment. It has been studied as a vehicle for pharmaceutical products such as topical steroids [8], as well as monotherapy for pruritic dermatoses [9]. Another benefit of aloe is that contact dermatitis to its application is rare, and it is generally well-tolerated.

- Oatmeal: *Avena sativa* is useful due to its colloidal protein and high mucilaginous content. It is commercially available as a bath-additive (Aveeno™), in soaps, and in emollients. Contact dermatitis is a possible side effect for patients who are allergic to oatmeal.

- Mind/body techniques: Several forms of breathwork, developed and taught by the Arizona Center for Integrative Medicine, can serve to allay the anxiety that often accompanies chronic pruritus and feeds into a vicious cycle. The overall goal is to slow down and deepen the breath.

  - 4-7-8 breath: Patients are counseled to breathe in for a count of 4, hold the breath for a count of 7, then breathe out for a count of 8. The ratios matter more than the speed of the breath, and this should be repeated for four cycles, twice daily.

- Square breathing: Patients are instructed to imagine that over two breath cycles (in, out, in, out) they are drawing the four sides of a square.
- "I am, at peace": With each inhale, the patient thinks, "I am," and with each exhale, "at peace."

Case Discussion This patient exhibited clear features of xerosis as a causative factor for his pruritus—In such cases, it is reasonable to first engage in a therapeutic trial of emollients and counseling on gentle skin care practices, prior to pursuing a full laboratory and malignancy screening workup. If these methods do not work, or if the review of systems points to another underlying etiology, then earlier testing is warranted.

He was given a list of mild non-soap cleansers, laundry soaps, and was counseled to avoid fabric softeners and scented dryer sheets. He was also advised to use lukewarm water and limit his showers to 10 min each, soaping (but not scrubbing) only his armpits/groin/feet. He was given a list of thick emollients to use BID, including those containing pure aloe, burdock, oatmeal and calendula (many are available at natural foods stores). Finally, he was educated about breathwork as a way of dispelling pruritus sensations while driving in his cab.

References

1. Burdock Root for Acne. Retrieved on 20 Jan 2014 from Livestrong.Com
2. Chan YS, Cheng LN, Wu JH, Chan E, Kwan YW, Lee S.M.Y, ... & Chan SW. A review of the pharmacological effects of Arctium lappa (burdock). Inflammopharmacology. 2011;19(5):245–54.
3. Farnsworth NR, Segelman AB. Hypoglycemic plants. Tile Till. 1971;57:52–6.
4. Bever BO, Zahnd GR. Plants with oral hypoglycaemic action. Q J Crude Drug Res. 1979;17:139–96.
5. Barnes J, Anderson LA, Phillipson JD. Herbal medicines. London: Pharmaceutical Press; 2002.

6. Panahi Y, Sharif MR, Sharif A, et al. A randomized comparative trial on the therapeutic efficacy of topical aloe vera and Calendula officinalis on diaper dermatitis in children. Scientific World Journal. 2012;2012:810234.
7. Akihisa T, Yasukawa K, Oinuma H, et al. Triterpene alcohols from the flowers of compositae and their anti-inflammatory effects. Phytochemistry. 1996;43(6):1255–60.
8. Davis RH, Parker WL, Murdoch DP. Aloe vera as a biologically active vehicle for hydrocortisone acetate. J Am Podiatr Med Assoc. 1991;81(1):1–9.
9. Syed TA, Ahmad SA, Holt AH, Ahmad SA, Ahmad SH, Afzal M. Management of psoriasis with Aloe vera extract in a hydrophilic cream: a placebo-controlled, double-blind study*. Trop Med Int Health. 1996;1(4):505–50.

Chapter 4
A 58 Year Old with Sun Damaged Skin

Jaimie B. Glick and Reena Rupani

Case Presentation

A 58-year-old white female presents to the office with complaints of wrinkles and light brown "sun spots" on her cheeks and forehead. The patient reports that people often mistake her for a much older woman. She admits to frequent sunbathing during the summer months until age 40 with little to no use of sunscreen and feels that her skin changes may be related to this prior sun exposure. She reports feeling overwhelmed by the number of over-the-counter anti-wrinkle creams and would like to know which cosmeceuticals are most effective and will truly help her appear her stated age.

J.B. Glick • R. Rupani (✉)
Department of Dermatology, SUNY Downstate Medical Center,
Brooklyn, NY, USA
e-mail: reena_rupani@yahoo.com

R.A. Norman, R. Rupani, *Clinical Cases in Integrative Dermatology*, Clinical Cases in Dermatology 4,
DOI 10.1007/978-3-319-10244-3_4,
© Springer International Publishing Switzerland 2015

Diagnosis Photoaging

Overview of Photoaging

Photoaging is defined as chronic cutaneous changes resulting from long-term exposure to ultraviolet (UV) light. Wrinkling is one of the most common features of skin photoaging and is caused by the accumulation of abnormal/damaged elastic fibers in the dermis. Other signs of photoaging include a dry, rough appearance to the skin as well as dark spots and uneven skin pigmentation (Fig. 4.1).

There has long been a societal demand for products that can halt or reverse the photoaging process. Consequently there are a tremendous number of over-the-counter remedies and services available to patients that claim to "reverse the signs of aging" and "reduce fine lines and wrinkles." Termed cosmeceuticals, these products are not regulated by the FDA, but can play an active role in skin health. Given the large number of products available, it is important for clinicians to distinguish between those that are beneficial and evidence-based from those that are not.

Pathogenesis

The ultraviolet spectrum is divided into UVA (400–315 nm), UVB (315–290 nm) and UVC (290–200 nm). Almost all of the UVC radiation is absorbed by the earth's atmosphere and essentially does not reach ground level. Both UVA and UVB contribute to photoaging with UVA probably playing a more substantial role in the aging process. UVA is better able to penetrate into the dermis as a result of its longer wavelength. Additionally, UVA is able to transmit through window glass resulting in sun exposure even while indoors or driving [1].

Reactive oxygen species (ROS) induced by UVA and UVB radiation leads to the activation of matrix metalloproteinases (MMPs), MMP-1, MMP-3 and MMP-9. MMPs cleave specific sites on collagens I and III leading to

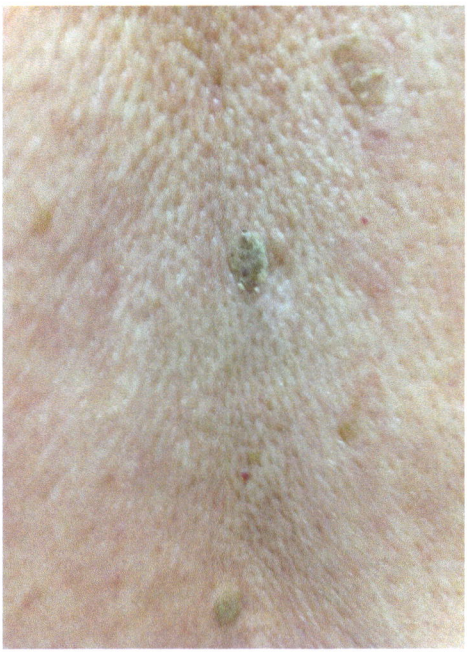

FIGURE 4.1 Dyschromia and loss of skin elasticity as seen in areas of chronic sun damage

collagen degradation. Collagen fibers are replaced by abnormal elastin fibers in the dermis (solar elastosis). Although less is known about the effects of UV radiation on the epidermis, there have been reports of epidermal atrophy leading to the obvious appearance of sebaceous glands and telangiectasias even without wrinkling [2].

Clinical Features

The effects of UV light vary based on skin phototype; patients with phototypes I and II are at increased risk of developing sun-related skin damage. The regions of the body predominately affected by photoaging are those most exposed to the sun, including the face, neck, upper chest, back, as well as the dorsum of the hands [2]. The clinical characteristics of photoaging in fair-skinned individuals include fine and coarse wrinkles, solar elastosis (thickening and yellowish discoloration of the skin), solar lentigines, and ephelides. Darker skinned patients can also have the previously mentioned findings but tend to present more commonly with seborrheic keratosis and pigmentary alterations [1]. Chronic sun exposure can also result in a leathery appearance to the skin and the development of telangiectasias. The loss of dermal collagen leads to skin fragility, and often patients will present with ecchymoses even after minor trauma—This is referred to as actinic purpura.

Treatment

As the term implies, photoaging is a direct result of chronic sun exposure. The most important factor in the treatment (and prevention) of photoaging is sun protection. UVB intensity is highest between the hours of 9 am and 3–4 pm. The sun protection factor (SPF) is used to measure a sunscreen's capacity to block UVB radiation. The SPF implies that sunscreen is applied to the body in an amount equivalent to 2 mg/cm^2, which is frequently much less than the amount applied by most users. It is recommended that sunscreen with an SPF of at least 30 be applied daily at least 20 min prior to sun exposure. Reapplication of sunscreen is important especially after exercise [2]. A recent in vitro study in France demonstrated that sunscreen protection of cells significantly reduced UVA-induced expression of matrix metalloproteinase-1, -3 and -9, which are the MMPs implicated in the collagen breakdown of photoaging [3].

Retinoids are comprised of synthetic and natural analogs of vitamin A. Retinoids bind to specific nuclear receptors and can modulate the expression of genes involved in cellular growth and differentiation. Tretinion and tazarotene are prescription retinoids that have been shown to improve wrinkling and uneven pigmentation by enhancing collagen synthesis, dispersing melanin and correcting the atypia associated with UV radiation. It takes about 3–6 months of use to see clinical improvement with topical retinoid applications [4]. Side effects such as skin irritation and peeling often occur but usually decrease over continued application.

Laser treatment is another option, and the ablative carbon dioxide (CO_2) laser is the gold standard for photorejuvenation. The CO_2 laser allows for significant skin tightening and wrinkle reduction. However, the ablative treatment often results in a prolonged postoperative course with persistent erythema and pigmentary changes. Newer nonablative laser treatments have been developed to combat these undesirable side effects.

However, laser treatments remain invasive procedures that are not desirable or cost effective for all patients. Other options for the treatment of photoaging skin include botulinum toxin injections, chemical peels, dermabrasion, rhytidectomy, blepharoplasty, and brow lifts. Furthermore, there are an overwhelming number of cosmeceuticals available, which are not regulated by the Food and Drug Administration (FDA) and can be misleading and confusing to patients. These will be the remaining focus of this chapter.

Cosmeceuticals

Cosmeceutical is a term coined by Albert Kligman, MD over two decades ago to refer to non-prescription topical products containing biologically-active ingredients designed to improve the function and appearance of the skin. Hydroxy acids (including alpha and beta) are among the most well-known cosmeceuticals and are frequently employed as peels for photodamaged skin as well as for the treatment of acne and rosacea. In addition to hydroxy acids there are a number of cosmeceuticals marketed as agents for the treatment and prevention of photoaging. Many of these products contain antioxidants that confer photoprotection by scavenging free radical oxygen species (ROS) and blocking UV-induced inflammatory pathways.

Vitamin C (ascorbic acid) is a water-soluble vitamin with antioxidant and anti-inflammatory properties found in many fruits and vegetables. In several in vitro and in vivo studies vitamin C has been shown to enhance dermal collagen synthesis and decrease collagen degradation and melanin formation. In a 12-week double-blind, split-face trial, topical application of vitamin C lead to significant improvement in photoaging scores and skin wrinkling. Additionally, histological evaluation of the skin treated with topical vitamin C showed increased collagen production [5]. In a study by Lin et al., a topical solution of 15 % L-ascorbic acid (vitamin C) and 1 % α-tocopherol (vitamin E) was found to be protective against erythema and sun burn cell formation after irradiation [6]. A later study showed that the plant antioxidant ferulic acid improved the chemical stability of the vitamin C and E solution as well as doubled its photoprotection ability [7].

Green tea is produced by steaming and drying the leaves of the tea plant, *Camellia sinensis*. This process does not require fermentation allowing the preservation of the teas polyphenolic compounds and its potent antioxidant properties. Epigallocathechin-3-gallate is the most abundant polyphenol present in green tea. In a recent study, the application of sunscreens containing 2–5 % green tea extract to human skin significantly reduced the expression of MMP-2 and MMP-9 [8]. In another study, skin biopsies of patients treated with both oral and topical green tea demonstrated significant improvement in elastic tissue content [9].

Pomegranate *(Punica granatum)* is a tree native to Asia commonly prepared as a juice, concentrate, jam or jelly. Pomegranate contains several polyphenols conferring its potent antioxidant effects [10]. The most abundant polyphenol present in *Punica granatum* is ellagic acid. In several studies, ingestion of an oral supplement containing 5 % ellagic acid increased sunscreen SPF by 25 %. In another study, UV irradiated human skin fibroblasts treated with *Punica granatum* extracts displayed increased synthesis of collagen and decreased expression of MMP-1 [11].

Soy *(Glycine max)* contains phosopholipids, essential fatty acids, vitamin E, and isoflavones and possesses both anti-oxidant and anti-inflammatory properties. Isoflavone extracts were shown to inhibit UVB-induced apoptosis and inflammation in both in vitro and in vivo studies [12]. Additionally, in a study of 65 women, twice daily application of a soy moisturizer was found to improve fine lines, skin tone, skin texture and overall appearance when compared to vehicle [13].

Shiitake mushroom (*Lentinula edodes*) extract contains the active ingredients eritadenine and L-ergothioneine conferring its anti-oxidant and anti-irritant effects. The cutaneous application of shiitake mushroom extracts is thought to be effective in the treatment of photoaging as it improves skin elasticity. In fact, natural shiitake complex has been shown to inhibit elastase in a dose dependent manner [14]. In a study by Miller et al., twice daily application of mushroom extract cleansing pads were found to have significant improvements in skin sallowness and tone, fine lines and irregular pigmentation [15]. It is important to note, however, that shiitake mushrooms when consumed raw can sometimes induce a dermatitis characterized by a linear distribution of erythematous papules and petechiae referred to as a flagellate erythema [16].

Resveratrol is a polyphenolic phytoalexin present in the skin and seeds of grapes, nuts, fruits and red wine. Recent studies have shown that topical application of resveratrol protects against UVB-induced skin damage in SKH-1 hairless mice [17]. Coffeeberry (*Coffea Arabica*) extract contains the polyphenols chlorogenic acid, quinic acid, ferulic acid and condensed proanthocyanidins and is another antioxidant thought to be effective in the prevention and treatment of photoaging, although evidenced-based data is lacking.

Peptides are short-chain amino acids sequences being utilized in many cosmeceutical products. Peptides are believed to enhance collagen production, decrease skin wrinkling and improve skin barrier function. Peptides can be divided into three categories: signal peptides, neuropeptides and carrier peptides. The cutaneous application of the signal peptide valine-glycine- alanine-proline-glycine has been shown to stimulate production of human dermal fibroblasts and reduce elastin [18]. In one open-label study of ten female patients, the application of a 5 % acetyl-hexapeptide-3 neuropeptide cream twice daily demonstrated improvement in periorbital wrinkles after 30 days of treatment [19]. In another study, oral supplementation with whey protein in melanin-possessing hairless mice inhibited the reduced elasticity and wrinkle formation associated with photoaging [20]. Furthermore, it is thought that priming of skin with peptides and growth factors prior to laser resurfacing treatments may enhance the laser effects as well as improve healing [18].

The topical retinoic acids tazarotene and tretinoin, discussed previously, are prescription medications and thus not classified as cosmeceuticals. However, there are a number of over the counter retinol/retinaldehyde preparations effective for the treatment of sun-damaged skin. In a small clinical trial, topical retinyl palmitate 2 % was found to be as effective as SPF 20 in preventing UVB-induced erythema and thymine dimer formation [21]. In a randomized double-blind, vehicle controlled study, 0.4 % retinol application improved fine wrinkles after 4 weeks of treatment. Biopsies of skin treated with the retinol showed increased collagen production [22]. The literature suggests retinaldehyde is the most effective of the retinoid-based cosmeceuticals. It is efficacious and well tolerated at a concentration of 0.05 % [23].

Discussion

In treating patients for photoaging a systematic approach is important. Morning treatments should include environmental protection with antioxidant and sunscreen containing products, whereas nightly skin care regimens should focus on tissue repair [18]. The patient above used a dermatologist-developed peptide-containing facial cleanser twice daily for 3 months. She was instructed to use a daily moisturizer containing vitamin C as well as SPF 30 or higher sunscreen. She began using tretinoin 0.05 % cream every other night and then increased treatment to nightly as skin irritation and redness improved. After 5 months, the patient reported noticeable improvement in her wrinkles and dark spots and plans to continue to use the treatment regimen.

References

1. Rünger AM. Ultraviolet light. In: Bolognia JL, Jorizzo JJ, Schaffer JV, editors. Dermatology. 3rd ed. Beijing: Elsevier; 2012. p. 1455–65. Chap. 37.
2. James WD, Berger TG, Elston DM. Dermatoses resulting from physical factors. In: Andrew's diseases of the skin: clinical dermatology. 11th ed. Elsevier Health Sciences; 2011. pp. 18–44 (Chap. 3).
3. Jean C, Bogdanowicz P, Haure MJ. UVA-activated synthesis of metalloproteinases 1, 3 and 9 is prevented by a broad-spectrum sunscreen. Photodermatol Photoimmunol Photomed. 2011;27:318–24.
4. Thielen AM, Saurat J. Retinoids. In: Bolognia JL, Jorizzo JJ, Schaffer JV, editors. Dermatology. 3rd ed. Beijing: Elsevier; 2012. p. 2089–103. Chap. 126.
5. Fitzpatrick RE, Rostan EF. Double-blind, half-face study comparing topical vitamin C and vehicle for rejuvenation of photodamage. Dermatol Surg. 2002;28:231–6.
6. Lin JY, Selim A, Shea CR. UV photoprotection by combination topical antioxidants vitamin C and vitamin E. J Am Acad Dermatol. 2003;48:866–74.
7. Lin FH, Lin JY, Gupta RD. Ferulic acid stabilizes a solution of vitamins C and E and doubles its photoprotection of skin. J Invest Dermatol. 2005;125:826–32.
8. Li YH, Wu Y, Wei HC, et al. Protective effects of green tea extracts on photoaging and photoimmunosuppression. Skin Res Technol. 2009;15:338–45.
9. Chiu AE, Chan JL, Kern DG, et al. Double-blinded, placebo-controlled trial of green tea extracts in the clinical and histologic appearance of photoaging skin. Dermatol Surg. 2005; 31:855–60.
10. Aslam MN, Lansky EP, Varani J. Pomegranate as a cosmeceutical source: pomegranate fractions promote proliferation and procollagen synthesis and inhibit matrix metalloproteinase-1 production in human skin cells. J Ethnopharmacol. 2006;103: 311–8.

11. Park HM, Moon E, Kim AJ, et al. Extract of Punica granatum inhibits skin photoaging induced by UVB irradiation. Int J Dermatol. 2010;49:276–82.
12. Chiu TM, Huang CC, Lin TJ, et al. In vitro and in vivo anti-photoaging effects of an isoflavone extract from soybean cake. J Ethnopharmacol. 2009;126:108–13.
13. Warren W, Nebus J, Leyden JJ. Efficacy of a soy moisturizer in photoaging: a double-blind, vehicle-controlled, 12-week study. J Drugs Dermatol. 2007;6:917–22.
14. Bowe W. Cosmetic benefits of natural ingredients: mushrooms, feverfew, tea and wheat complex. J Drugs Dermatol. 2013; 12(Suppl):s133–6.
15. Miller D, Wallo W, Leyden JJ. Clinical evaluation of exfoliating cleansing pads containing a complex of mushroom extracts for improving photoaged skin. Poster presented at 67th annual meeting of the American Academy of Dermatology. San Francisco, 6–10 Mar 2009.
16. Adriano AR, Acosta ML, Azulay DR, et al. Shiitake dermatitis: the first case reported in Brazil. An Bras Dermatol. 2013;88:417–9.
17. Afaq F, Adhami VM, Ahmad N. Prevention of short-term ultra-violet B radiation-mediated damages by resveratrol in SKH-1 hairless mice. Toxicol Appl Pharmacol. 2003;186:28–37.
18. Reszko AE, Berson D, Lupo MP. Cosmeceuticals: practical applications. Dermatol Clin. 2009;27:401–16.
19. Blanes-Mira C, Clemente J, Jodas G, et al. A synthetic hexapep-tide (Argireline) with antiwrinkle activity. Int J Cosmet Sci. 2002;24:303–10.
20. Kimura Y, Sumiyoshi M, Kobayashi T. Whey peptides prevent chronic ultraviolet B radiation-induced skin aging in melanin-possessing male hairless mice. J Nutr. 2014;144(1):27–32.
21. Antille C, Tran C, Sorg O, et al. Vitamin A exerts a photoprotec-tive action in skin by absorbing UVB radiation. J Invest Dermatol. 2003;121:1163–7.
22. Kafi R, Kwak HS, Schumacher WE, et al. Improvement of natu-rally aged skin with vitamin A (retinol). Arch Dermatol. 2007;143:606–12.
23. Babamiri K, Nassab R. Cosmeceuticals: the evidence behind the retinoids. Aesthet Surg J. 2010;30:74–7.

Chapter 5
A 46 Year Old African American Woman with White Spots

Raman Madan and Reena Rupani

Case Presentation

A 46 year old African American woman presents for evaluation of white spots on both her arms that have been spreading. She says that she first noted the spots 2 years ago. There were initially two spots on her right arm and three on her left arm. They have combined and become larger. Before this, she says she had perfect skin and did not even have acne as a teenager. She denies any pain or trauma to the areas. She says she has tried to scrub the spots when showering but it has not helped. She has also applied several name brand lotions to the spots daily. While her skin has remained moisturized, her lesions have not improved. She is very self-conscious about the lesions and is afraid that it may be "some type of cancer."

R. Madan • R. Rupani (✉)
Department of Dermatology, SUNY Downstate Medical Center, Brooklyn, NY, USA
e-mail: reena_rupani@yahoo.com

R.A. Norman, R. Rupani, *Clinical Cases in Integrative Dermatology*, Clinical Cases in Dermatology 4, DOI 10.1007/978-3-319-10244-3_5, © Springer International Publishing Switzerland 2015

She tries to wear long sleeve shirts to avoid having her arms seen because she feels it makes her look deformed. She is upset because the weather is getting warm but she is embarrassed to wear short sleeve t-shirts. She does feel she gained weight over the last several months and becomes fatigued very quickly. She denies any fever, chills, headache, shortness of breath, palpitations, or excessive sweating. She feels her menses have been less frequent. She has no allergies and does not take any medications.

The patient is married and has two children. She works as a swim instructor. She is now embarrassed to wear a bathing suit and often wears a sweatshirt to cover her arms. She says she used to exercise three times a week for 1 h but can hardly go once a week for half an hour because she gets tired. In an attempt to stop gaining weight, she has changed her diet from ordering take out to eating salads and lean meat. She drinks alcohol socially and has never smoked.

On examination, her blood pressure is 120/80 and her HR is regular in the low 60s. She is in no acute distress and moderately obese. She has bilateral depigmented patches on her forearms. On the right arm, there is amelantoic skin with irregular borders extending from the wrists to the elbows. The borders show the depigmented patch expanding into normally pigmented skin. On her left arm, there is one large amelanotic patch with discrete margins that is beginning to overlap with several 1–2 mm punctate macules extending up her forearm. The patient also has a 3 cm hypopigmented patch on her left shin. There are no findings on her right leg.

Differential Diagnosis

1. Vitiligo
2. Chemical Leukoderma
3. Postinflammatory hypomelanosis
4. Pityriasis (tinea) versicolor
5. Tuberous Sclerosis
6. Piebaldism

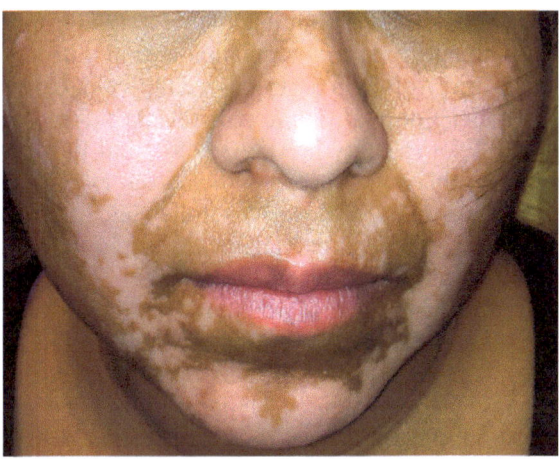

FIGURE 5.1 Depigmented macules of vitiligo

Vitiligo: Vitiligo is a chronic depigmenting disorder that is characterized by a complete absence of melanocytes in the epidermis. It presents initially with white macules that can enlarge and eventually affect the entire skin ([1]; Fig. 5.1) While the disease can start at any time, vitiligo most commonly begins in childhood or young adulthood with peak ages of onset between 10 and 30 years [2]. Several pathogenic mechanisms are hypothesized and include autoimmunity, oxidant-antioxidant mechanisms, transepidermal melanocytorrhagy, neural mechanisms and intrinsic defects of melanocytes [3]. Vitiligo can be classified many ways including focal, segmental, or most commonly, generalized. Given the cosmetic concerns, this disease can cause severe psychological distress, especially in those with darker skin [4].

Chemical Leukoderma: Chemical leukoderma, or occupational vitiligo, is caused by exposure to agents such as phenolic germicides, thiols, catechols, mercatoamines, and several quinines. Typically depigmented patches will only occur in areas where skin has contact with chemical agents [5].

Postinflammatory hypomelanosis: Postinflammatory hypomelanosis is a very common skin disorder that occurs more often in dark skinned individuals. Psoriasis, seborrheic dermatitis, atopic dermatitis, sarcoidosis, lichen sclerosis, pityriasis versicolor, and lupus can all produce this secondary hypomelanosis. Decreased pigmentation most often occurs following inflammation but complete depigmentation can occur after severe atopic dermatitis or discoid lupus [5].

Pityriasis (tinea) versicolor: Pityriasis (tinea) versicolor normally presents with multiple oval to round patches or thin plaques with mild, fine scale. Patients can be hyper or hypopigmented. Hypopigmentation is secondary to inhibitory effects of dicarboxylic acids on melanocytes as well as decreased tanning secondary to the ability of the malassezia yeast to filter sunlight [5].

Tuberous Sclerosis: Tuberous Sclerosis Complex is an autosomal dominant disorder that can present with a white macule most often on the trunk in addition to hamartomas in multiple organs. Hypomelanotic macules can be lance-ovate and confetti shaped. This is usually due to decreased size and poor development of melanosomes [5].

Piebaldism: Piebaldism is rare autosomal dominant disorder due to abnormal migration of melanoblasts. Clinically there are patches of depigmented skin with hyperpigmented borders most often on the mid-forehead, neck, anterior trunk, and mid-extremities. A white forelock is a common finding. The disorder is stable and permanent but patients generally have a normal lifespan [5].

Further Workup Wood's lamp examination is useful for lightly pigmented patients. Skin biopsy for histopathology and melanin stains can be used to confirm the diagnosis in difficult cases [5]. On further history, the patient denies any occupational hazards or exposure to chemicals. She does not give a family history of similar symptoms. The patient endorses constipation. There is a documented weight gain of 25 lb over 2 years. A serum level of thyroid stimulating hormone is found to be above the upper limit of normal.

Diagnosis Vitiligo

Discussion Vitiligo comes in multiple forms. The most common form is described as discrete amelanotic milky-white macules and patches ranging from 5 mm to 5 cm or greater surrounded by normal skin. Trichrome vitiligo is a variant that has three colors (white, light brown, dark brown). Inflammatory vitiligo is a variant with an elevated erythematous potentially pruritic margin. Vitiligo ponctue is characterized by multiple small confetti-like discrete amelanotic macules occurring on normal or hyperpigmented skin [6].

Most patients with vitiligo are otherwise healthy, although associated autoimmune endocrinopathies can occur in some individuals. The strongest association is thyroid disease, therefore a screening with review of systems and possible TSH is indicated. There are also studies showing association of vitiligo with diabetes mellitus and cases of vitiligo associated with Addison's disease, gonadal failure, and pernicious anemia [5, 7].

In our patient, above, we see an association with hypothyroidism. She has the most common form of vitiligo, which is progressive. The components of the diseases seem to be associative rather than causative. Therefore each issue should be dealt with separately.

There is no cure for vitiligo. A conventional treatment algorithm would include:

- Two month trial of mid-high potency steroids for focal/limited disease
- Topical calcipotriene daily to help increase efficacy of steroids
- Tacrolimus (0.1 %) ointment to cosmetically sensitive areas or genital skin, twice daily

- PUVA (phototherapy): topical application of 8-methoxy-psoralen to affected areas followed by controlled ultraviolet A (UVA) exposure for focal disease, and methoxsalen capsules 2 h before UVA in systemic disease.
- Narrow band UVB twice weekly (may take up to 200 treatments) [8, 9]
- Surgical therapy such as minigrafting for limited, stable disease unresponsive to therapies [10]
- Total depigmentation for severe disease with 20 % monobenzyl ether of hydroquinone applied twice daily for 9–12 months [11, 12]

An integrative treatment algorithm can include substances which are applied topically, ingested, or available commercially. They can be used alone or as supplements to conventional therapies.

Topical integrative approaches are as follows.

- Coconut oil for the strong antioxidant activity [13].
- Black cumin or the seeds of Nigella sativa—efficacy is due to its immunomodulatory effect [13]
- Bavachi (Psoralia carylifolia), a psoralen derivative, to help induce pigmentation [14].
- Polypodium leucotomos, a type of fern native to the tropical and subtropical regions of the Americas when combined with PUVA [15]
- Piperine, the major alkaloid of black pepper, stimulates melanocyte proliferation when combined with UV radiation [16].
- Amino acid L-phenylalanine reduces Langerhans cells present in lesional skin [17].
- Chinese cupping: providing suction over the skin to induce blisters on the thigh whose roofs are subsequently used for epithelial grafts [18]
- Dead Sea Therapy: patients spend several weeks between late February and mid-November [19]

    - High salt concentration, high $MgCl_2$ concentration of water, and solar radiation are reasons for efficacy
    - Pseudocatalase cream can be added [20]

Oral therapies which have showed benefit are as follows.

- Ginkgo biloba 40 mg PO three times a day or 60 mg PO twice a day [21]

  - Anti-inflammatory, immunomodulatory, antioxidant, and anxiolytic effects [22]
  - Cheap, relatively few side effects

- Vitamin E (antioxidant) 900 IU/day in combination with PUVA [23]
- Antioxidants: Vit B12, Vit C, Folic Acid, Vit A 20,000 IU, Vit C 1,000 mg, Zinc 15 mg, Selenium 50 µg, Magnesium 2 mg, CoQ10 75 mcg, and pygnogenol 1 mg [24]
- Herbs: Liquid extract of Acacia catechu bark, Psoralea corylifolia leaves with psorlanes [25]

  - Hyperemia caused by psoralen increases melanin producing activity in skin
  - Monitor for hepatotoxicity

- Chinese mixture of "Xiaobai" 160 mL, orally daily [26]

  - Contains 30 g walnut, 10 g red flower, 30 g black sesame, 30 g black beans, 10 g zhi bei fu ping, 10 g lu lu tong, 5 plums

Several commercial products are available as well.

- Anti-vitiligo®: contains Coconut Oil, Psoralea corylifolia, Black cumin, and Barberry root [27]
- Vitilo© lotion: apply a thin layer two to three times to the affected area of skin, wait roughly 30 min, or until the lotion dries and then expose the area to sunlight for 5–20 min. Side effects include itching which can be treated with coconut oil [28].

  - Composed of 4 % Bavachi (Psoralia carylifolia), 1 % Karanja (Pongamia glabra), 2 % Neem (Azadirachta indica), 2 % Manjistha (Rubia cordifolia), 1 % Haldi (Curcuma longa), 1 % Amba Haldi (Curcuma amada), 2 % Raktachandan (Pterocarpus Santalinum), 1 % Vacha (Acorus calamus), and 4 % processed Jasad Bhasma (ZINC OXIDE)

- Bonzastrong© lotion: similar to Vitilo© lotion [29]
- Kalawalla® (polypodium leucotomos): works by increasing lymphocyte levels and regulating the CD4/CD8 levels to a normal ratio [13]

  - Taken orally: 120 mg of P. leucotomos extract and 280 mg of P. leucotomos rhizome
  - Pruritus is a common side effect

- Melagenina Plus©: initially extracted from human placenta tissue and now other animal placental tissues [30].

  - The cream should be applied and then the affected skin should be exposed to 15 min of natural sunlight
  - Thought to work by stimulating the proliferation and differentiation of immature melanocytes and melanoblasts [31]

Support groups can be important for patients who are embarrassed and become isolated because of their vitiligo.

- Vitiligo Support International: http://www.vitiligo support.org/
- Vitiligo Friends: http://www.vitiligofriends.org/

The patient was initially treated with topical steroids but she had minimal response to the therapy. She did not feel she had the time for phototherapy given her work and family life. She joined Vitiligo Friends, an online support group, and spoke with members who had success with alternative therapies. It was explained that despite the paucity of strong evidence-based studies, the potential therapeutic benefit of many of these treatments should not be overlooked. Locating some of the recommended herbs was difficult, so she was started on Gingko biloba 60 mg twice a day. She also continued her medium-potency topical steroid 2 weeks per month compounded with petroleum jelly. Six months into her treatment course, her disease stopped progressing but lesions have not fully improved. However, after starting the Gingko she reports feeling less anxious about her appearance. She has begun experimenting with special makeup lines (Dermablend™). She has also set up an appointment with an endocrinologist to manage her hypothyroidism.

References

1. Wolff K, Johnson RA, Suurmond D. Section 13: Pigmentary disorders – vitiligo. Fitzpatrick's color atlas & synopsis of clinical dermatology. 6th ed. New York: McGraw-Hill; 2009.
2. Wolff K, et al. Fitzpatrick's dermatology in general medicine. 7th ed. New York: McGraw Hill; 2007. p. 616–21.
3. Kopera D. Historical aspects and definition of vitiligo. Clin Dermatol. 1997;15(6):841–3.
4. Halder RM, Taliaferro SJ. Vitiligo. In: Wolff K et al., editors. Fitzpatrick's dermatology in general medicine. 7th ed. New York: McGraw-Hill; 2008. Chap. 72.
5. Bolognia JL, Jorizzo JL, Rapini R. Dermatology. 2nd ed. St. Louis: Mosby Elsevier; 2008. p. 1023–48.
6. Gauthier Y. The importance of Koebner's phenomenon in induction of vitiligo vulgaris lesions. Eur J Dermatol. 1995;5:704–8.
7. James WD, et al. Andrews' diseases of the skin: clinical dermatology. London: Saunders; 2011.
8. Westerhof W, Nieuweboer-Krobotova L. Treatment of vitiligo with UV-B radiation vs topical psoralen plus UV-A. Arch Dermatol. 1997;133(12):1525–8.
9. Scherschun L, Kim JJ, Lim HW. Narrow-band ultraviolet B is a useful and well-tolerated treatment for vitiligo. J Am Acad Dermatol. 2001;44(6):999–1003.
10. Gupta S, Honda S, Kumar B. A novel scoring system for evaluation of results of autologous transplantation methods in vitiligo. Indian J Dermatol Venereol Leprol. 2002;68(1):33–7.
11. Mosher DB, Parrish JA, Fitzpatrick TB. Monobenzylether of hydroquinone. A retrospective study of treatment of 18 vitiligo patients and a review of the literature. Br J Dermatol. 1977;97(6):669–79.
12. Bolognia JL, LaPia K, Somma S. Depigmentation therapy. Dermatol Ther. 2001;14:29–34.
13. Tahir MA, et al. Current remedies for vitiligo. Autoimmun Rev. 2010;9(7):516–20.

14. Panda AK. The medico historical perspective of vitiligo (Switra). Bull Indian Inst Hist Med Hyderabad. 2005;35(1):41–6.
15. Reyes E, Jaén P, de las Heras E, Carrión F, Alvarez-Mon M, de Eusebio E, et al. Systemic immunomodulatory effects of polypodium leucotomos as an adjuvant to PUVA therapy in generalized vitiligo: a pilot study. J Dermatol Sci. 2006;41:213–16.
16. Faas L, et al. In vivo evaluation of piperine and synthetic analogues as potential treatments for vitiligo using a sparsely pigmented mouse model. Br J Dermatol. 2008;158(5):941–50.
17. Felsten ML, Alikhan A, Petronic-Rosic V. Vitiligo: A comprehensive overview – Part II: treatment options and approach to treatment. J Am Acad Dermatol. 2011;65(3):493–514.
18. Awad SS. Chinese cupping: a simple method to obtain epithelial grafts for the management of resistant localized vitiligo. Dermatol Surg. 2008;34(9):1186–92.
19. Czarnowicki T, et al. Dead Sea climatotherapy for vitiligo: a retrospective study of 436 patients. J Eur Acad Dermatol Venereol. 2011;25(8):959–63.
20. Schallreuter KU, et al. Rapid initiation of repigmentation in vitiligo with Dead Sea climatotherapy in combination with pseudocatalase (PC-KUS). Int J Dermatol. 2002;41(8):482–7.
21. Parsad D, Pandhi R, Juneja A. Effectiveness of oral Ginkgo biloba in treating limited, slowly spreading vitiligo. Clin Exp Dermatol. 2003;28(3):285–7.
22. Szczurko O, et al. Ginkgo biloba for the treatment of vitilgo vulgaris: an open label pilot clinical trial. BMC Complement Altern Med. 2011;11:21.
23. Akyol M, Celik VK, Ozcelik S, Polat M, Marufihah M, Atalay A. The effects of vitamin E on the skin lipid peroxidation and the clinical improvement in vitiligo patients treated with PUVA. Eur J Dermatol. 2002;12:24–6.
24. Rojas-Urdaneta JE, Poleo-Romero AG. Evaluation of an antioxidant and mitochondria-stimulating cream formula on the skin of patients with stable common vitiligo. [Spanish]. Investigacion Clinica. 2007;48:21–31.
25. Teschke R, Bahre R. Severe hepatotoxicity by Indian ayurvedic herbal products: a structured causality assessment. Ann Hepatol. 2009;8(3):258–66.
26. Szczurko O, Boon HS. A systematic review of natural health product treatment for vitiligo. BMC Dermatol. 2008;8:2.
27. Antivitiligo.com [Internet]. Pakistan: TrueHerbal laboratories; c2009 [updated 22 Apr 2009; cited 12 Dec 2013]. http://www.antivitiligo.com/

28. Vitilo Lotion [Internet]. India: Elder healthcare; c2013 [updated 2013;cited 12 Dec 2013].http://www.elderhealthcare.in/vitilo.aspx-

29. BonzaStrong [Internet]. Mukesh medical hall; c2009 [updated 2013; cited 12 Dec 2013]. http://mukeshmedicalhall.com/contact-us.html

30. Nordlund JJ, Melagenina HR. An analysis of published and other available data. Dermatologica. 1990;181(1):1–4.

31. Zhao D, et al. Melagenine modulates proliferation and differentiation of melanoblasts. Int J Mol Med. 2008;22(2):193–7.

Chapter 6
A 48 Year Old Male Alcoholic with Multiple Plaques

Reena Rupani

Case Presentation

A 48 year old male alcoholic is brought in by ambulance to an urban emergency department with symptoms of alcohol withdrawal. He has presented on several occasions within the last 12 months for the same symptoms of tremor, tachycardia, diaphoresis, and a clear history of "running out of booze." His past medical history is otherwise significant for hypertension diagnosed on a previous admission, for which he is non-compliant with medication outside the hospital. He denies any medication allergies.

He lives with his girlfriend in a rent-subsidized studio apartment and works construction for a living. He admits to drinking on a nightly basis, often with friends, but denies tobacco or other toxic ingestions. He rides a motorcycle without a helmet and engages in several other high-risk behaviors, such as occasional unprotected female sexual intercourse (non-monogamous) and tattoos. His diet consists mostly of fast food and sandwiches, with very little fresh fruit or vegetable intake.

R. Rupani
Department of Dermatology, SUNY Downstate Medical Center, Brooklyn, NY, USA
e-mail: reena_rupani@yahoo.com

R.A. Norman, R. Rupani, *Clinical Cases in Integrative Dermatology*, Clinical Cases in Dermatology 4, DOI 10.1007/978-3-319-10244-3_6,
© Springer International Publishing Switzerland 2015

On examination, he is a stocky Caucasian male in mild distress, shaking, but able to converse freely. He is tachycardic to 120 bpm and his skin feels clammy. He points to his ankles, saying that they have been very itchy lately, and are actually causing him quite a bit of distress although unrelated to his current presentation. He has never taken off his socks to show a doctor before.

Skin examination of his ankles reveals multiple purple, polygonal, flat-topped violaceous papules, some with an overlying white lacy scale, and many with an excoriated surface. A through skin exam then reveals similar lesions on the glans penis, and a few lacy white plaques in his bilateral buccal mucosa. He has 10/10 onychodystrophy of the fingernails, which he has previously attributed to his work in construction. A few dorsal pterygia are noted on several fingernails. He exhibits trachyonychia of the toenails as well. He is also diffusely covered on the upper and lower extremities with multiple tattoos, a mixture of professional and home-applied varieties.

Differential Diagnosis

1. Eczematous dermatitis
2. Syphilis/STIs
3. Lichen planus
4. Morsicatio buccarum (oral mucosa)

   Eczematous dermatitis—While eczema can present as pruritic papular lesions, involvement of the mucosal areas and nails would not be consistent with this diagnosis.

   Syphilis/STIs—The patient does give a history of high-risk sexual behaviors, and syphilis can involve both cutaneous and mucosal skin. If he is engaging in receptive oral sex, one could consider involvement of the oropharynx. Further testing would clarify. Syphilitic lesions are not typically pruritic, however.

   Lichen planus—The typical appearance of lichen planus (LP) is pruritic purple polygonal planar papules (Fig. 6.1). Wickham's striae is the term to describe the lacy white scale that can manifest on top of the lesions. LP is sometimes painful, particularly when involving the genital and oral mucosa, as well as nails.

Morsicatio buccarum (oral mucosa)—This diagnosis refers to the whitish bite line that can be seen on buccal mucosa, and is typically bilateral, and associated with cheek biting. This would not explain the rest of his physical findings, however.

Further Workup While the patient is hospitalized for his withdrawal symptoms, a dermatology consult is placed and skin biopsy obtained. Liver function tests reveal a transaminitis, and hepatitis C antigen is positive. He is found to be HIV and RPR negative and other laboratory values are within normal limits, including hepatitis B serology.

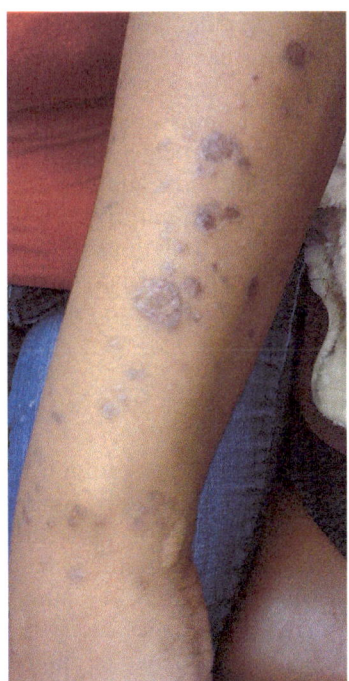

FIGURE 6.1 Purple polygonal planar papules of lichen planus

Diagnosis Lichen planus

While the precise etiology of lichen planus is unknown, an immunological mechanism involving CD8 + –mediated destruction of basal keratinocytes has been proposed, initiated by either an endogenous or exogenous antigenic stimulus. As described above, lesions are typically purplish in color, itchy, and may exhibit a phenomenon of koebnerization. Various clinical manifestations of LP include annular, hypertrophic, atrophic, ulcerative, bullous, linear, and pigmented. Additionally, LP of the scalp is termed lichen planopilaris, and is a form of scarring alopecia. There is an increased risk of developing squamous cell carcinoma in chronic lesions of oral LP [1]. Mucosal LP refers to that affecting the lining of the gastrointestinal tract (mouth, pharynx, esophagus, stomach, anus), larynx, and other mucosal surfaces including the genitals, peritoneum, ears, nose, bladder and conjunctiva of the eyes.

Several studies have looked at the association between LP and hepatitis C, with mixed results. A systematic review from 2010 found that lichen planus patients have a significantly higher risk than controls of being hepatitis C virus (HCV) seropositive, and a similar odds ratio of having lichen planus was found among HCV patients [2]. However, subgroup analysis revealed that the strength of this association varied geographically. Certainly a lichen planus patient with positive risk factors for HCV should undergo serological testing.

Conventional Treatment Strategies

Topical approaches—High-potency topical steroids are typically first-line treatment, and can be compounded in adhesive vehicles (Orabase™) for application to mucosal surfaces [3]. Non-steroidal anti-inflammatory medications such as topical tacrolimus 0.1 % ointment can also be applied twice daily to non-mucosal surfaces. Additionally, viscous lidocaine compounded with diphenhydramine and a calcium carbonate-based antacid (Maalox™) can be used as a mouth rinse prior to meals for pain relief in oral LP.

Systemic approaches—Phototherapy in the form of narrow-band ultraviolet B can be useful in some forms of cutaneous lichen planus [4], but in patients with darker skin types there is a higher risk of post-inflammatory hyperpigmentation.

Oral prednisone in doses of 0.5–1 mg/kg tapered slowly over 6–8 weeks can be used in severe or erosive disease. Intramuscular steroids injections (triamcinolone 40 mg/cc) can also confer several weeks of remission at a time. Unfortunately, disease relapse with steroid taper is common [3], and the longer time course of treatment increases the myriad risks of steroid side effects.

Oral acitretin in doses of 10–50 mg/day, systemic methotrexate 5–25 mg/week, oral cyclosporine 3–5 mg/kg divided BID, and other immunosuppressants such as mycophenolate mofetil are employed for widespread or recalcitrant disease, but do require periodic laboratory monitoring for systemic side effects.

Additionally, referral to other services such as gastroenterology or otolaryngology should be directed by a patient's review of systems.

Integrative Treatment Strategies

Lifestyle modifications—Given the increased risk of squamous cell carcinoma in oral lichen planus, patients should be counselled on decreasing alcohol consumption as well as smoking cessation [5].

Dietary modifications—For patients with oral lichen planus, counseling on the avoidance of hard/sharp-edged foods, spicy foods, and highly acidic foods and beverages is an important component of pain management. One could also propose that the general benefit of high fruit and vegetable/antioxidant consumption would be significant, although one particular prospective cohort study that investigated such a relationship found that fruit consumption decreased the risk of oral premalignant lesions, while vegetable consumption had no consistent association [5]. Still, general principles of wound healing dictate that sufficient protein, zinc, and vitamin C consumption, at the very least, would be beneficial in ulcerative or erosive lesions.

Supplements and Herbs

- Purslane: Oral purslane (*Portulaca oleracea*), a botanical medicine, was studied at a dose of 235 mg/day for treatment of oral lichen planus, and found to be significantly effective over placebo in a randomized double-blind placebo controlled trial [6].
- Aloe vera: Topical application of aloe vera gel has also demonstrated evidence of symptom relief and reduced disease burden in oral LP [7].
- Curcumin: A randomized, double-blind, placebo-controlled clinical trial was recently conducted in which individuals with oral lichen planus were treated with 6,000 mg/day of curcuminoid product in three divided doses [8]. With a good safety profile, curcuminoids were found to ameliorate symptoms of oral LP.

Mind/Body Approaches

- Hypnosis: The precise pathophysiological mechanism of hypnosis is unknown; however, many of its effects are thought to be derived through autonomic regulation [9]. Hypnosis is particularly effective at decreasing inflammation and associated inflammatory discomfort and is therefore specifically applicable to inflammatory skin disorders such as lichen planus [10]. Additional benefits are relaxation, diminishing social stress, and improving an individual's attitude about the disease state.
- Yoga/meditation: As LP can manifest with symptoms of both itch and pain, the emotional distress can be quite significant. Yoga and meditation are two potential avenues of mind control and sublimation of chronic pain [11].
- Breathwork: Rapid shallow breathing often accompanies (and exacerbates) severe pain or itch, so deep and measured

breathing are also effective strategies for symptom control and stress reduction. The 4-7-8 breath, pioneered by Dr. Andrew Weil of the University of Arizona Center for Integrative Medicine, is one such technique. Patients are instructed to breathe in for a count of 4, hold for a count of 7, and breathe out for a count of 8, repeating four cycles, twice daily.

The patient was treated for alcohol withdrawal, and discharged with a prescription for triamcinolone 0.1 % ointment to use on his cutaneous LP lesions. He was additionally recommended to take milk thistle extract (Silybum marianum) for its hepatoprotective effects [12], and given planned follow-up with hepatology and dermatology. Given his many socioeconomic and lifestyle challenges, a measured approach to care was employed. He was generally disinterested in mind-body techniques, but was given a handout describing various breathwork strategies, with the idea that he may be able to take a few minutes out during his lunch break to "center" himself. He found this concept interesting. Of greatest importance, he was willing to join alcoholics anonymous, and expressed interest in reducing his alcohol intake.

References

1. Gandolfo S, Richiardi L, Carrozzo M, Broccoletti R, Carbone M, Pagano M, Merletti F. Risk of oral squamous cell carcinoma in 402 patients with oral lichen planus: a follow-up study in an Italian population. Oral Oncol. 2004;40(1):77–83.
2. Lodi G, Pellicano R, Carrozzo M. Hepatitis C virus infection and lichen planus: a systematic review with meta-analysis. Oral Dis. 2010;16(7):601–12.
3. Usatine R, Tinitigan M. Diagnosis and treatment of lichen planus. Am Fam Physician. 2011;84(1):53–60.
4. Habib F, Stoebner PE, Picot E, Peyron JL, Meynadier J, Meunier L. Narrow band UVB phototherapy in the treatment of widespread lichen planus. Annales de dermatologie et de vénéréologie. 2005;132(1):17.

5. Maserejian NN, et al. Prospective study of fruits and vegetables and risk of oral premalignant lesions in men. Am J Epidemiol. 2006;164(6):556–66.
6. Agha-Hosseini F, et al. Efficacy of purslane in the treatment of oral lichen planus. Phytother Res. 2010;24(2):240–4.
7. Choonhakarn C, et al. The efficacy of aloe vera gel in the treatment of oral lichen planus: a randomized controlled trial. Br J Dermatol. 2008;158(3):573–7.
8. Chainani-Wu N, et al. High-dose curcuminoids are efficacious in the reduction in symptoms and signs of oral lichen planus. J Am Acad Dermatol. 2012;66(5):752–60.
9. Shenefelt P. Hypnosis in dermatology. Arch Dermatol. 2000;136:393–9.
10. Shenefelt PD. Relaxation, meditation, and hypnosis for skin disorders and procedures. In: De Luca BN, editor. Mind-body and relaxation research focus. Hauppauge: Nova; 2008. p. 45–63.
11. Vallath N. Perspectives on yoga inputs in the management of chronic pain. Indian J Palliat Care. 2010;16(1):1.
12. Pradhan SC, Girish C. Hepatoprotective herbal drug, silymarin from experimental pharmacology to clinical medicine. Indian J Med Res. 2013;137(2):423.

Chapter 7
A 30 Year Old Woman with a Red Face

Jaimie B. Glick and Reena Rupani

Case Presentation

A 30-year-old female presents to the office complaining of redness of her face. The patient reports that over the last few months her face is often flushed and she sometimes felt a stinging sensation of her bilateral cheeks. The symptoms are worse after she spends time outside playing tennis or drinking alcohol. She also notices that for several minutes after application of certain facial cleansers and lotions her face would burn. More recently she developed prominent blood vessels along the sides of her nose.

She works for a financial company and admits her job is stressful as she works long hours and often has to go into the office on weekends. She regularly has in-person meetings

J.B. Glick • R. Rupani (✉)
Department of Dermatology, SUNY Downstate Medical Center,
Brooklyn, NY, USA
e-mail: reena_rupani@yahoo.com

R.A. Norman, R. Rupani, *Clinical Cases in Integrative Dermatology*, Clinical Cases in Dermatology 4,
DOI 10.1007/978-3-319-10244-3_7,
© Springer International Publishing Switzerland 2015

with clients and is embarrassed of her facial flushing which has been occurring more and more frequently. The patient reports several attempts at dieting, as she would like to lose about 10 lb. She tries to avoid foods high in carbohydrates and sugar. She does enjoy spicy foods and often cooks with jalapeno peppers and chili powder. She admits to occasional alcohol use and usually drinks about three to four alcoholic beverages per week, usually on the weekends. She exercises about three times per week usually running on the treadmill or in the park by her home.

On examination, she is well-appearing and thin. Her cheeks display symmetrical erythematous patches and there are some telangiectasias of her bilateral nasal ala. There is no evidence of comedones, papules, or pustules on her face. She is very concerned with the new changes in her skin and would like treatment.

Differential Diagnosis

1. Rosacea
2. Acne Vulgaris
3. Seborrheic dermatitis
4. Chronic Actinic damage

Rosacea: Rosacea comprises a number of signs and symptoms including flushing, persistent facial erythema, telangiectasias, inflammatory papules and pustules, facial edema, phymatous changes and ocular inflammation. In 2002, an expert committee of the National Rosacea Society published a report classifying rosacea into four major subtypes: erythematotelangiectactic rosacea, papulopustular rosacea, phymatous rosacea and ocular rosacea. The erythematotelangiectactic form presents with persistent centrofacial erythema, flushing, skin sensitivity and occasionally telangiectasias. Papulopustular rosacea is characterized by a centrofacial distribution of transient erythematous papules or pustules with individual lesions usually lasting a few

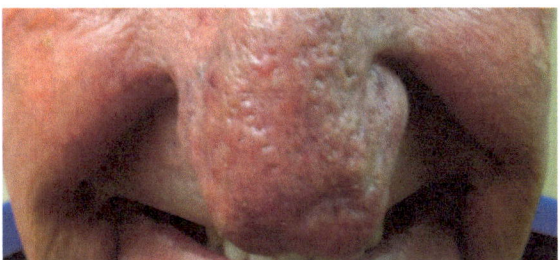

FIGURE 7.1 Edema and fibrosis as a severe manifestation of phymatous rosacea

weeks. Phymatous rosacea leads to skin thickening, irregular surface changes and edema. Rhinophyma is the most common presentation of phymatous rosacea and results from hypertrophy of the sebaceous glands of the skin (Fig. 7.1). Ocular rosacea consists of a variety of signs and symptoms including redness, dryness, tearing, burning, itching or stinging as well as a foreign body sensation, light sensitivity, blurred vision and crusting of the eyelids. Ocular rosacea may occur on its own or in association with the cutaneous findings of rosacea.

Acne Vulgaris: Acne can often be confused with the papulopustular form of rosacea. However, acne differs from rosacea in that patients with rosacea do not develop comedones, and the pathogenesis of rosacea is primarily inflammatory without much involvement of Propionibacterium acnes.

Seborrheic dermatitis: Seborrheic dermatitis can present as facial erythema, and often accompanies rosacea as a co-morbid condition; however, patients with pure seborrheic dermatitis usually present with a greasy, yellowish scale and frequently have involvement of the nasolabial folds and eyebrows.

Chronic Actinic damage: Patients with skin changes related to chronic sun exposure usually show evidence of damage on extrafacial skin including the ears, chest and neck helping to distinguish the condition from rosacea.

Further Work Up   There is no histological or laboratory marker of rosacea. The diagnosis requires the presence of one or more of the following characteristics concentrated on the central portion of face: flushing (transient erythema), non-transient erythema, papules and pustules, and telangiectasias. Persistent erythema is the most common finding in rosacea and some dermatologists believe the diagnosis of rosacea can be made simply by the presence of persistent erythema of the central face lasting for at least 3 months. It is also essential to rule out other causes of facial flushing and erythema including polycythemia vera, connective tissue disorders, carcinoid syndrome and mastocytosis.

Diagnosis   Rosacea (Erythematotelangietactic Rosacea)

Discussion

The treatment of rosacea is long-term as the condition is a chronic one with frequent recurrences and flaring. Additionally, treatment varies with each subtype of rosacea. The patient discussed above has erythematotelangiectatic (EMT) rosacea. The treatment of EMT rosacea includes gentle skin care and regular application of sunscreen with ultraviolet A and ultraviolet B protection. In 2013, the FDA approved brimonidine topical gel 0.33 % (Mirvaso™, Galderma Laboratories) for facial erythema in rosacea patients 18 years or older. Brimonidine is an alpha-adrenergic agonist that constricts dilated blood vessels and reduces the erythema and facial flushing of rosacea. Laser therapy is often effective for the treatment of telangiectasias. Many topical treatments used to treat papulopustular rosacea such as metronidazole or azelaic acid may be ineffective or even exacerbate EMT rosacea.

Several topical products have been FDA-approved for the treatment of rosacea and seem to be particularly effective in the papulopustular form. These topical products include the gel, cream and lotion formulations of 0.75 % metronidazole applied twice daily and 1 % metronidazole cream or gel applied once daily. Azelaic acid 15 % gel applied twice daily as well as multiple formulations of the sulfacetamide 10 %-sulfur 5 % are also FDA-approved for the treatment of rosacea. Systemic treatments for rosacea include oral antibiotics as well as isotretinoin [1]. Doxycycline 40 mg (controlled release) daily is FDA-approved for rosacea and is thought to be effective due to its anti-inflammatory properties. The treatment of phymatous rosacea is difficult and often requires surgical excision or laser therapy. Ocular rosacea should be treated with eyelid hygiene and artificial tears. Topical or systemic antibiotics may be necessary and patients should be referred to an ophthalmologist.

In an otherwise healthy, young patient it is unnecessary to perform any further diagnostic work up. Rosacea is a clinical diagnosis made by history and physical examination.

Conventional treatment options for EMT rosacea would include the following:

- Facial cleansing with lukewarm water and gentle cleansers
- Daily Sunscreen with SPF of 30 or higher
- Gentle moisturizers and emollients to improve barrier function
- Avoidance of exfoliating agents, physical scrubbing, astringents and toners
- Refraining from products containing alcohol, eucalyptus oil, menthols, and fragrances
- Cosmetic coverage with water-soluble powder containing light green or yellow pigment to neutralize redness
- Avoidance of triggers including hot environments and sun exposure
- Topical oxymetazoline
- Topical brimonidine gel 0.33 %
- Pulse dye laser and intense pulse light device for treatment of erythema and telangiectasias

An integrative approach to treatment would encompass the above methods particularly focused on gentle skin care techniques. A number of botanical and over-the-counter products with anti-oxidant and anti-inflammatory properties may also be beneficial as adjunctive treatments.

– Niacinamide is the biologically active amide of vitamin B3 with anti-inflammatory and anti-oxidant effects. Use of a niacinamide-based moisturizer may enhance stratum corneum barrier function and skin hydration improving the irritant symptoms in rosacea.
– Licochalcone A has been shown to improve the erythema in patients with facial redness and was even comparable to treatments with topical metronidazole and azelaic acid.
– Green tea is derived from the leaves of *Camellia sinensis* through a process of steam drying avoiding fermentation and preserving the polyphenolic compounds of the leaves. Green tea contains anti-oxidant and anti-inflammatory effects and has been shown to decrease ultra violet-induced erythema and DNA damage.
– Chrysanthellum indicum (C. indicum) is a plant-based extract containing phenylpropenoic acids, flavonoids and saponosids, with effects on vascular wall permeability and capillary resistance.
– Purified feverfew (Tanacetum parthenium) may reduce erythema and redness, and is available commercially (Eucerin™ Redness Relief, Beiersdorf AG).
– Aloe vera gel or cream and colloidal oatmeal have soothing effects on inflamed and irritated skin.

Dietary Modifications are important to therapy:

– Spicy foods can increase the basal metabolic rate exacerbating facial erythema and flushing.
– Reducing the consumption of alcohol and onions may help, as both have vasodilatory effects. Skin affected by rosacea has shown elevated levels of vascular endothelial growth factor (VEGF) and lymphatic endothelial markers suggesting stimulation of vascular and lymphatic endothelial cells. There is also evidence for increased blood flow in lesional skin in patients with rosacea.
– Patients should be encouraged to keep a journal logging their rosacea triggers. There are a number of foods and/or

facial products that may exacerbate an individual's signs and symptoms.

Stress reduction with a focus on the relationship between the mind and body:

- Biofeedback: This technique trains patients to exert control over involuntary autonomic responses to stimuli. Patients may over time be able to modulate responses to skin temperature thus reducing the facial erythema associated with hot environments and sun exposure.
- Hypnosis: Neurogenic mediators of inflammation have important effects on vasodilation and may play key role in the pathogenesis of rosacea. Hypnosis is thought to regulate autonomic functions such as blood flow as well as affect the neurohormonal system and may prove beneficial in rosacea patients. Additionally, the relaxation state induced by hypnosis may in itself improve facial erythema and flushing.
- Support groups: As rosacea is a disorder primarily of the facial skin it can be very distressing to patients. Referral to online or local support groups is important for patients with this chronic condition. The National Rosacea Society (www.rosacea.org) contains an abundance of information on the condition as well as skin care tips and cosmetic recommendations.

The patient was told to discontinue use of harsh facial cleaners as she was regularly washing her face with a benzoyl peroxide over the counter facial cleanser and using a salicylic acid-based astringent. Instead, she switched to a gentle soap-free facial cleanser and no longer scrubs with a washcloth after rinsing. She was instructed to moisturize with a morning facial lotion containing SPF 30 and a niacinamide-containing facial lotion at bedtime. The patient was also counselled to avoid spicy foods and alcohol. She was encouraged to keep a journal logging other possible triggers. At a 3 month follow up visit, she reported significant improvement in her facial erythema. However, she reported no improvement in the telangiectasias and is considering laser therapy.

Bibliography

1. Baldwin HE. Oral therapy for rosacea. J Drugs Dermatol. 2006;5:16–21.
2. Chen JH, Tsai SJ, Chen HI. Welsh onion (Allium fistulosum L.) extracts alter vascular responses in rat aortae. J Cardiovasc Pharmacol. 1999;33:515–20.
3. Crawford GH, Pelle MT, James WD. Rosacea I. Etiology, pathogenesis, and subtype classification. J Am Acad Dermatol. 2004;51:327–41.
4. Del Rosso JQ, Baldwin H, Webster G. American Acne & Rosacea Society rosacea medical management guidelines. J Drugs Dermatol. 2008;7:531–3.
5. Draelos ZD, Ertel K, Berge C. Niacinamide-containing facial moisturizer improves skin barrier and benefits subjects with rosacea. Cutis. 2005;76:135–41.
6. Emer J, Waldorf H, Berson D. Botanicals and anti-inflammatories: natural ingredients for rosacea. Semin Cutan Med Surg. 2011;30:148–55.
7. Martin K, Sur R, Lienel F, et al. Parthenolide-depleted Feverfew (Tanacetum parthenium) protects skin from UV irradiation and external aggression. Arch Dermatol Res. 2008;300:69–80.
8. National Rosacea Society. Rosacea triggers survey. http://www.rosacea.org. Accessed 26 Nov 2013.
9. Powell FC, Raghallaigh SN. Rosacea and related disorders. In: Bolognia JL, Jorizzo JJ, Schaffer JV, editors. Dermatology. 3rd ed. Beijing: Elsevier; 2012. p. 561–9. Chap. 37.
10. Rigopoulos D, Kalogeromitros D, Gregoriou S, et al. Randomized placebo-controlled trial of a flavonoid-rich plant extract-based cream in the treatment of rosacea. J Eur Acad Dermatol Venereol. 2005;19:564–8.
11. Shenefelt PD. Biofeedback, cognitive-behavioral methods, and hypnosis in dermatology: is it all in your mind? Dermatol Ther. 2003;16:114–22.
12. Shenefelt PD. Hypnosis in dermatology. Arch Dermatol. 2000;136:393–9.
13. Somboonwong J, Thanamittramanee S, Jariyapongskul A, et al. Therapeutic effects of aloe vera on cutaneous microcirculation and wound healing in second degree burn model in rats. J Med Assoc Thai. 2000;83:417–25.
14. Weber TM, Ceilley RI, Buerger A, et al. Skin tolerance, efficacy and quality of life of patients with red facial skin using a skin

care regimen containing Licochalcone A. J Cosmet Dermatol. 2006;5:227–32.

15. Wilkin J, Dahl M, Detmar M, et al. Standard classification of rosacea: report of the National Rosacea Society expert committee on the classification and staging of rosacea. J Am Acad Dermatol. 2002;46:584–7.

Chapter 8
A 25 Year Old Woman with Excess Sweating

Reena Rupani

Case Presentation

A 25-year-old woman presents for evaluation of excess sweating of her armpits. She notes that for the past 3 years, she has been experiencing a chronic underarm dampness that is not well-controlled by any over-the-counter antiperspirant (she states that she has "tried them all"). She describes her problem as sweaty but not malodorous. She states that she often has to change her blouse in the middle of the day. She is frequently embarrassed in public situations and has been increasingly avoiding friends and even loved ones, which subsequently makes her feel anxious and depressed. She denies any other symptoms including fevers, weight loss, palpitations, headaches, or tremors. Her past medical history is negative and she denies any medications or allergies. She takes a daily multivitamin but denies any other vitamins or supplements. Her menses are monthly and normal.

R. Rupani
Department of Dermatology, SUNY Downstate Medical Center, Brooklyn, NY, USA
e-mail: reena_rupani@yahoo.com

R.A. Norman, R. Rupani, *Clinical Cases in Integrative Dermatology*, Clinical Cases in Dermatology 4, DOI 10.1007/978-3-319-10244-3_8, © Springer International Publishing Switzerland 2015

63

She works as a paralegal and lives alone. She has a few close friends, but does not socialize much because of her embarrassment. She exercises once or twice per week in the gym and relaxes by reading mystery novels. Her diet consists of mostly vegetables and fish, but she admits to frequent caffeine (three cups of coffee per day). She does not drink alcohol or smoke cigarettes.

On examination, her blood pressure is 110/60 and her pulse is regular in the 1970s. She is well-developed and well-nourished. Her axillae bilaterally are visibly damp but not malodorous. She does not exhibit excess sweating of any other body sites. She does not exhibit any tremors.

Differential Diagnosis

Primary hyperhidrosis—Hyperhidrosis is defined as perspiration in excess of what is needed for physiologic thermoregulation. Primary focal hyperhidrosis, the most common type, is excess regional sweating that is idiopathic in nature, and with localization following the distribution of eccrine sweat glands, which are most densely concentrated in the face, axillae, palms and soles (Fig. 8.1). In primary hyperhidrosis, the cause is not thought to be due to the sweat gland or duct itself (which is typically histologically and functionally intact) but instead is an abnormal or exaggerated central response to normal emotional stress.

Secondary hyperhidrosis—Secondary hyperhidrosis is excessive sweating due to an underlying condition. There are a multitude of such secondary etiologies, including a medication side effect, hyperthyroidism, carcinoid syndrome, pheochromocytoma, or a paraneoplastic phenomenon. This form of hyperhidrosis is typically generalized.

Further Workup   Laboratory analysis for thyroid function is within normal limits. A chest x-ray is negative for masses or adenopathy. Further, the patient's review of symptoms and physical examination do not support an underlying pathology. She does not take any medications or supplements.

Diagnosis   Primary focal hyperhidrosis

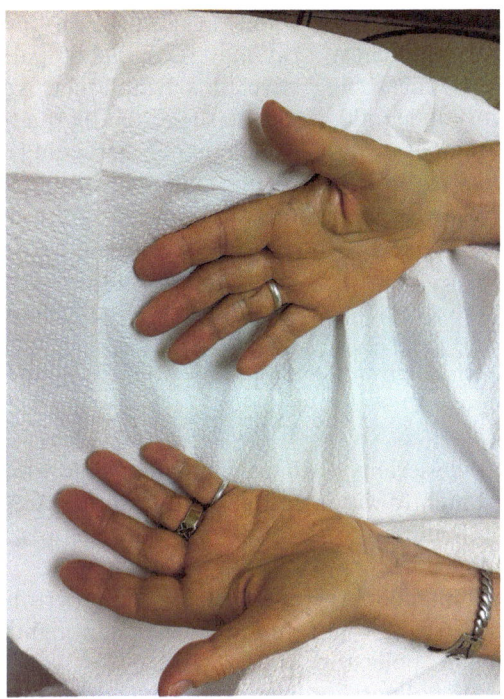

FIGURE 8.1 Diffuse sweating of the palms

Discussion

Hyperhidrosis is a common presenting complaint, and typical distributions include palms/soles, axillae, face, and other regional foci.

For secondary hyperhidrosis, treatment involves the identification and elimination of underlying causative factors. Common medication culprits would include cholinesterase inhibitors, selective serotonin reuptake inhibitors, opioids and tricyclic antidepressants. Basic labs including thyroid function studies should be performed, and if guided by the review of symptoms, may also include a workup for metabolic by-products suggestive of a carcinoid tumor or a pheochromocytoma (urinary 5-HIAA, and 24 h urinary catecholamines and metanephrines, respectively). If the patient is female, LH/FSH studies could suggest the onset of meno-pause. A routine chest x-ray may reveal adenopathy or an intrathoracic mass suggestive of a lymphoma. Additional cancer workup should, again, be suggested by the review of systems. Age-appropriate malignancy screening such as colonoscopy and mammography should also be up to date.

In a typical case of an otherwise young, healthy individual, as outlined above, the most likely diagnosis is primary focal hyperhidrosis, which we term idiopathic but may involve a decreased response threshold to emotional and chemical stimuli.

Conventional treatment options would follow the algo-rithm below:

- Topical desiccants such as aluminum chloride (20 %) applied nightly with a cotton ball for up to 6 weeks (lim-ited by irritation), then two to three times per week as needed.
- Topical anticholinergic agents such as glycopyrrolate, com-pounded 0.5–2 % in solution and applied nightly with a cotton ball applicator.
- Oral anticholinergic agents (glycopyrrolate, oxybutynin, propanthelene)
- Oral beta-blockers (such as propranolol)
- Iontopheresis
- Non-invasive microwave based technology (MiraDry™)
- Onabotulinum toxin A injected in region of excess sweat (40–50 units per axillary vault)
- Surgical removal of glands or regional sympathectomy as a last resort

An integrative approach to treatment would likely include many of the above measures, but would also touch on the mind-body component of the condition:

- Biofeedback: This technique trains patients to control bodily processes (in response to stress triggers) that are normally involuntary, such as skin temperature or mois-ture level, using galvanic skin response to measure electrical conductance. The goal is to learn to control these responses without the help of monitoring.

– Acupuncture: Stimulation of certain anatomic sites via insertion of fine needles can decrease over-excitation of nerve endings and therefore regulate sweat production.

– Hypnosis: Hypnosis may exert its effects through regulation of autonomic functions such as blood flow and neurohormonal modulation, but also essentially produces a state of relaxation.

– Psychotherapy: Counseling may prove beneficial in patients with a marked emotional component to their disease. Anxiety and depression do not appear to cause primary focal hyperhidrosis, but can certainly develop subsequently, or these conditions can concomitantly exacerbate each other creating a negative feedback loop.

Dietary modifications may also play an adjunctive therapeutic role:

– Reducing the intake of caffeine

– Reducing the amount of "heat" in the diet: Spicy foods and alcohol, which increase basal metabolic rate and cause vasodilation (respectively), can exacerbate sweating. Similarly, onions are vasodilatory, and consumption should be minimized while trying to control hyperhidrosis. Even though garlic does not affect sweating per se, the odor can be transmitted into sweat, thereby increasing the patient's distress.

Measures to target stress relief can be helpful:

– Botanicals—The dietary introduction of herbs such as lemon balm, sage, and ashwagandha can have adaptogenic and calming effects.

– Exercise—Increasing the amount of daily cardiovascular exercise to at least 30 min (five times per week) can boost endorphins, and while thermal sweating would naturally increase with exercise, the overall improvement in mood might decrease the anxiety that stems from and contributes to hyperhidrosis, thereby breaking a negative feedback loop.

- Journaling—Literature suggests a highly therapeutic role for written reflection and journaling, which can either be reviewed periodically with patients, or can be purely private, depending on preferences.
- Support groups—Referral to online or local support groups (International Hyperhidrosis Society: www.sweathelp.org) is very important for patients who are feeling isolated and withdrawn.

The patient was treated with topical glycopyrrolate solution, which provided insufficient relief, and so she elected to proceed with a series of injections of Onabotulinum toxin A (she was able to obtain insurance coverage for the procedure). She was not interested in oral medication or aggressive surgical approaches, but she was willing to make some dietary/lifestyle modifications (cutting back on caffeine, increasing her exercise). An English major in college, she also enjoyed the idea of therapeutic journaling and has begun a diary of daily stressors and joys.

Bibliography

1. Chen JH, et al. Welsh onion (Allium fistulosum L.) extracts alter vascular responses in rat aortae. J Cardiovasc Pharmacol. 1999;33(4):515–20.
2. Cheshire Jr WP, Fealey RD. Drug-induced hyperhidrosis and hypohidrosis. Drug Saf. 2008;31(2):109–26.
3. Consumer Lab Web Site. http://www.consumerlab.com. Accessed 20 Apr 2012.
4. Ellis J. Hyperhidrosis diet tips to stop excessive sweating. Web Site. http://www.prlog.org/10224407-hyperhidrosis-diet-tips-to-stop-excessive-sweating.html. Accessed 7 Mar 2012.
5. Freedberg I, et al. Fitzpatrick's dermatology in general medicine. 6th ed. New York: McGraw-Hill; 2003.
6. Pennebaker JW. Telling stories: the health benefits of narrative. Lit Med. 2000;19(1):3–18.
7. Ruchinkskas RA, et al. The relationship of psychopathology and hyperhidrosis. Br J Dermatol. 2002;147(4):733–5.

8. Schlereth T, et al. Hyperhidrosis—causes and treatment of enhanced sweating. Dtsch Arztebl Int. 2009;106(3):32–7.
9. Shenefelt P. Hypnosis in dermatology. Arch Dermatol. 2000;136:393–9.
10. Shenefelt PD. Biofeedback, cognitive-behavioral methods, and hypnosis in dermatology: is it all in your mind? Dermatol Ther. 2003;16(2):114–22.
11. Wang WZ, Zhao L. Acupuncture treatment for spontaneous polyhidrosis. J Tradit Chin Med. 2008;28(4):262–3.

Chapter 9
A 29 Year Old Man with Patchy Hair Loss

Reena Rupani

Case Presentation

A 29-year-old man presents to a dermatologist for complaints of recent hair loss in several patches on the back of his scalp. He describes that the hair seems to have fallen out "overnight" and was noticed by his girlfriend about 1 month ago. He denies any itching or pain in the area, and has not tried any treatments. His past medical history is negative, but his family history is positive for hypothyroidism and diabetes. He denies any medications or medical allergies, only taking the occasional multi-vitamin, or acetaminophen over the counter. He denies any recent major illnesses or particularly stressful events in his life.

He works as a fashion photographer and is therefore quite conscious of his appearance. So far, he has been able to cover his hair with a baseball cap or a hat, but is concerned that the spots seem to be progressing in size and number. He generally takes good care of his skin, and has a twice daily routine of cleansing followed by moisturizing. He describes his life as somewhat stressful, mostly because of professional obligations

R. Rupani
Department of Dermatology, SUNY Downstate Medical Center,
Brooklyn, NY, USA
e-mail: reena_rupani@yahoo.com

R.A. Norman, R. Rupani, *Clinical Cases in Integrative Dermatology*, Clinical Cases in Dermatology 4,
DOI 10.1007/978-3-319-10244-3_9,
© Springer International Publishing Switzerland 2015

and travel, but does not generally feel overwhelmed. He tries to exercise daily, and eats a diet consisting mostly of fish and vegetables. He is currently not sexually active, but has been in monogamous heterosexual relationships in the past, and always used condoms for protection. He is very motivated to take care of his health, and is open and amenable to "any and all approaches" to healing his scalp.

On physical exam, he is thin and tall, with normal vital signs and in no acute distress. On the occipital scalp there are three discrete 2–3 cm areas of non-scarring alopecia, with patent follicular ostia, and no erythema. There are a few grey hairs growing within the center of each patch (he otherwise has dark brown hair). On dermoscopic exam, several "exclamation point" hairs are noted at the edges of the lesions.

Differential Diagnosis

Alopecia areata—Affecting approximately 2 % of the population, alopecia areata is thought to be an autoimmine process leading to non-scarring hair loss of scalp, beard, or any other hair-bearing region of skin (Fig. 9.1). More advanced forms are termed alopecia totalis and universalis. When localized, the disease is often self-limiting, with resolution over 1–2 years and occasional relapses. Hairs can turn grey either immediately before falling out, or can appear grey on regrowth prior to resuming normal hair color. Tapered hairs noted on magnified exam are called "exclamation point hairs." As an autoimmune process, there is some association with thyroid dysfunction; patients sometimes will also give a history of antecedent stress prior to disease development ("hair turning grey overnight").

Trichotillomania—This term describes self-induced hair loss either from direct pulling, twirling, or other manipulation, and can be performed either consciously or unconsciously by the patient. Often a manifestation of anxiety or obsessive-compulsive disorder, trichotilloma-

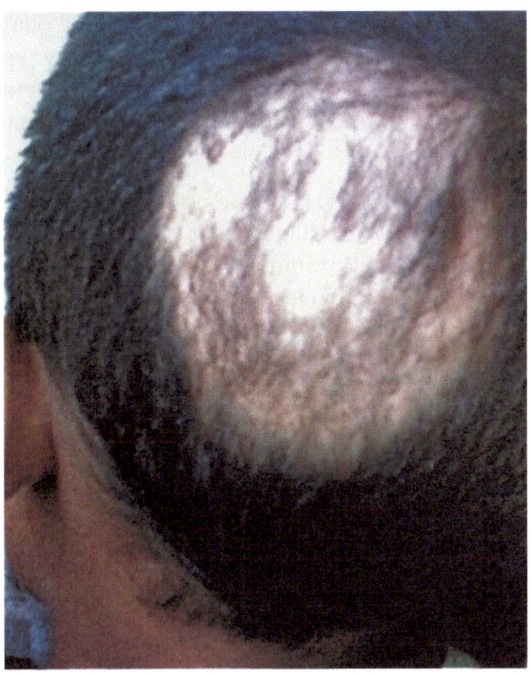

FIGURE 9.1 Focal non-scarring alopecia of the scalp

nia is typically focal, areas are not completely devoid of hair, and residual hairs are broken and of different lengths.

Telogen effluvium—Telogen effluvium refers to the sudden diffuse shedding that occurs, often following severe stress or a systemic insult such as major illness, childbirth, or surgery. Hair loss is generally non-focal.

Androgenetic alopecia—Also known as male or female pattern baldness, a combination of hormones and genetics play a causative role in androgenetic alopecia. In men, gradual thinning occurs typically over the vertex, bitemporal, and frontal scalp, whereas in women thinning begins over the top of scalp and partline, preserving the frontal hairline.

Syphilis—Classically described as "moth eaten," patchy hair loss can be a clinical manifestation of secondary syphilis. A careful review of systems, screening for risk factors, and confirmatory blood work can aid in the diagnosis if suspected.

Further Workup   A TSH is performed and found to be within normal limits. The diagnosis of alopecia areata is made by clinical history and examination; however, a scalp punch biopsy (sent for horizontal and vertical sectioning) could give confirmation, if needed, and would typically show inflammation around the base of the follicle in a "swarm of bees" configuration.

Diagnosis   Alopecia areata

Conventional Treatment Options

- **Intralesional steroid injections:** Typically the mainstay of therapy for alopecia areata, this treatment involves injecting the scalp (at the level of the reticular dermis) with dilute triamcinolone acetonide, typically in the strengths of 2.5–5 mg/cc mixed in normal saline (placed in depots of 0.1 cc each, spaced apart by approximately 1 cm, to cover the whole affected area). The maximum amount to be injected over the whole scalp in a single session should not exceed 3 cc of 5 mg/cc strength. Injections should be repeated at intervals every 4–6 weeks. If the steroid is placed too deep, i.e., within the subcutaneous fat, there is a higher likelihood of cutaneous atrophy.
- **Topical steroids:** High-potency (class 1) topical steroids applied to affected areas twice daily for 4–6 weeks can be an initial treatment option for pediatric patients, those with a needle aversion, or those in whom hair appears to have already started to regrow. Caution must be exercised to avoid cutaneous atrophy, although the scalp is typically more resilient to topical steroid use.

- **Topical squaric acid:** Squaric acid dibutylester and diphen-cyprone are topical contact sensitizers that are applied to the scalp in varying concentrations in different regimens, in order to induce and maintain an allergic contact derma-titis of affected areas of the scalp, as a form of immuno-therapy. Response rates can vary from 17 to 100 %, depending on the duration and extent of disease.
- **Topical retinoids:** Topical retinoids (tretinoin, bexarotene) have been shown in some studies, as well as anecdotally, to help with hair regrowth. The mechanism is not well-char-acterized but may include t-cell apoptotic pathways.
- **Topical anthralin:** Also used for psoriasis, anthralin cream or ointment can be applied in both short- and long-contact regimens, generating scalp irritation and hair growth.
- **Oral therapies:** Both pulsed systemic steroids and metho-trexate are treatment options for patients with moderate to severe alopecia, totalis or universalis. Use can be limited by toxicity and/or side effects.

Integrative Treatment Options

Botanical approaches

- **Raspberry ketones:** An aromatic compound contained in red raspberries (*Rubus idaeus*), a .01 % concentra-tion was applied to wild-type mice and was found to increase dermal levels of insulin-like growth factor I (IGF-I). Further, in a human trial, 50 % of study sub-jects with alopecia areata experienced hair growth after 5 months of daily application [1].

Supplements

- **Isoflavones/soy:** Isoflavones are phytoestrogens that, similarly to raspberry ketones, stimulate the release of calcitonin gene-related peptide which subsequently increases IGF-I expression and hair growth. In rat studies, dietary soy was found to have dose-dependent protective effect on hair follicles, and lower rates of alopecia areata development [2].

Mind-body approaches

- Yoga/meditation: There can be significant emotional distress associated with alopecia areata, but so, too, is stress thought to worsen the disease. Yoga and meditation are two potential avenues of mind control and sublimation [3].
- Breathwork: The 4-7-8 breath, pioneered by Dr. Andrew Weil of the University of Arizona Center for Integrative Medicine, is one technique for autonomic balancing and stress reduction. Patients are instructed to breathe in for a count of 4, hold for a count of 7, and breathe out for a count of 8, repeating four cycles, twice daily.

Anti-inflammatory diet: The Anti-Inflammatory Diet™, developed by Dr. Andrew Weil, reflects the belief that certain foods cause or combat systemic inflammation [4]. The goal of this eating plan is not weight loss, but instead a more balanced and healthy approach to food. The ratio of pro-inflammatory omega 6 fatty acids to anti-inflammatory omega 3 fatty acids is approximately 40:1 in the typical Western diet, whereas an ideal ratio is closer to 3:1. The direct benefit in alopecia areata is theoretical, but grounded in the concept of an autoimmune/inflammatory etiology.

Cosmetic approaches: There are various cosmetic and camouflage approaches to masking the hair loss, starting from (at the simplest level) working with a stylist to physically hide the hairless patches, to a more advanced approach using synthetic keratin fibers, which electromagnetically cling to the hair shaft and scalp; unfortunately, these products only last until the next hair washing. In cases of extensive alopecia areata of the scalp (patchy or totalis), some patients may chose to shave the head entirely. Locks of Love™ is an organization that provides human hairpieces to financially disadvantaged individuals under the age of 21 suffering from long-term medical hair loss.

Counseling: As with any disorder where there is a physically visible component, referral for counseling and supportive therapy may be helpful, and the subject should be broached with patients. The National Alopecia Areata Foundation has a useful website (www.naaf.org) and may allow patients to connect with others who are similarly afflicted via a virtual online community.

Case Discussion   The patient was treated with intralesional steroid injections monthly for 3 months, and elected to pursue several mind-body approaches to stress reduction for general overall wellness. He began attending yoga classes weekly, and also incorporated a 10 min meditative session with some focused breathwork upon waking daily. He was recommended to explore the National Alopecia Areata Foundation website. Six months later, his hair had completely regrown.

References

1. Harada N, Okajima K, Narimatsu N, Kurihara H, Kakagata N. Effect of topical application of raspberry ketone on dermal production of insulin-like growth factor-I in mice and on hair growth and skin elasticity in humans. Growth Horm and IGF Res. 2008;18:335–44.
2. McElwee KJ, Niiyama S, Freyschmidt-Paul P, Wenzel E, Kissling S, Sundberg JP, Hoffman R. Dietary soy oil content and soy-derived phytoestrogen genistein increase resistance to alopecia areata onset in C3H/HeJ mice. Exp Dermatol. 2003;12:30–6.
3. Vallath N. Perspectives on yoga inputs in the management of chronic pain. Indian J Palliat Care. 2010;16(1):1.
4. Weil A. Anti-inflammatory diet pyramid. http://www.drweil.com/drw/u/ART02995/Dr-Weil-Anti-Inflammatory-Food-Pyramid.html. Accessed 20 Mar 2012.

Chapter 10
An 8 Year Old Child with Recalcitrant Atopic Dermatitis

Reena Rupani

Case Presentation

An 8-year-old child presents to the office with her mother for evaluation of recalcitrant atopic dermatitis. She has had eczema since the age of 3, currently has a diagnosis of mild intermittent asthma, and seasonal allergies to pollen and ragweed. She has been managed by her primary care doctor with mild topical steroids (1 and 2.5 % hydrocortisone) as needed, but this is no longer sufficient to control her symptoms. She is primarily bothered by itching, which is worse at night and not very responsive to oral diphenhydramine. She also feels that her skin is more red and flaky than before.

Her current skincare regimen includes bathing daily in warm water for 20 min with unscented soap and a loofah sponge, followed by shea butter application to her skin after drying off with a towel. Her mother washes her clothes in scented baby laundry detergent, and then uses fabric softener.

R. Rupani
Department of Dermatology, SUNY Downstate Medical Center, Brooklyn, NY, USA
e-mail: reena_rupani@yahoo.com

R.A. Norman, R. Rupani, *Clinical Cases in Integrative Dermatology*, Clinical Cases in Dermatology 4, DOI 10.1007/978-3-319-10244-3_10, © Springer International Publishing Switzerland 2015

The patient is a third grade student who likes to read and does well in school. She has a close group of friends, but feels limited in play sometimes by her asthma, which can be exercise-induced. She is also increasingly embarrassed by her skin, and says there is a boy in her class who calls her "Itchy Scratchy". She lives with her mother and older brother, but spends alternate weekends at her father's home where there are smokers in the house. Neither household has pets, but there are old carpets in her father's house, according to the patient's mother.

She does not have any other medical problems, and her medications include an albuterol inhaler used as needed, as well as the hydrocortisone as mentioned above. She is not allergic to any medications but does have an allergy to fish and eggs. Her diet typically consists of breakfast cereals in the morning, a sandwich and chips with juice for lunch, granola bar and milk for an after-school snack, and either chicken or beef with rice and vegetables for dinner. Her mother notes that her skin seems to flare when she eats peanut butter, although the patient does not have a peanut allergy.

On examination, she is a thin child in no acute distress. Large ill-defined erythematous plaques with overlying white scale are distributed over her cheeks, trunk, and extremities, sparing the genital region. The plaques on her cheeks exhibit some yellow crusting.

Diagnosis   Atopic Dermatitis

Further Workup   None indicated at this time.

Discussion

Atopic dermatitis can afflict young and old, but is most commonly a presenting complaint to pediatricians (Fig. 10.1). There are a multitude of available conventional therapies, mostly in the form of topical steroids and immunomodulators, and yet there is a great deal of work remaining to be done in clarifying disease pathogenesis and improving treatment.

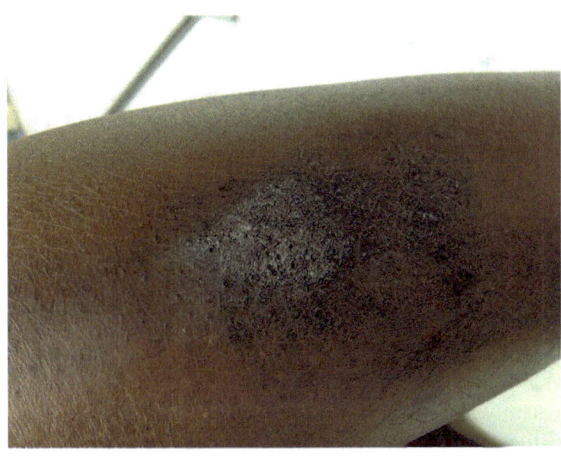

Figure 10.1 Ill-defined inflamed scaly plaques as typically seen in atopic dermatitis

Conventional Treatment Options

– Gentle skin care: A fundamental component of disease management is counseling patients on proper skin care—that is, the use of fragrance-free soaps and laundry detergents (avoiding fabric softeners); limiting baths to once daily in lukewarm water for no more than 10 min; avoiding the use of loofah sponges and washcloths, using only hands to apply soap (focusing on armpits, groin, feet); applying thick cream or ointment-based emollients to wet skin immediately after bathing.

– Topical/systemic steroids: Typically, mid- to high-potency topical steroids may be required for 1–2 weeks at a time, with twice daily application to the body (low potency steroids are preferred for sensitive areas such as face, axillae, and groin). Potential side effects with long-term continuous use include skin atrophy, striae, and steroid acne. Systemic steroids are generally not preferred due to the high risk of rebound disease, as well as increased propensity towards adverse effects.

- Topical immunomodulators: Topical non-steroidal immunomodulators such as tacrolimus and pimecrolimus have earned a major place in the therapeutic armamentarium, given their good safety profile and tolerability. However, there is a black box warning attached to these medications, and cost is prohibitive without insurance coverage.
- Antibiotics/antibacterials: Plaques of eczema are known to carry staph aureus as a colonizer (which can worsen the disease and increase sensation of itch) so treatment should also aim to decrease this colonization, either via topical/systemic antibiotics where indicated, or measures such as twice weekly bleach baths (one-fourth cup of bleach added to a whole tub of warm water, soak for 10 min).
- Antihistamines: Controlling itch is of major importance in atopic dermatitis management, since scratching can worsen the clinical appearance of the skin. Antihistamines are not reliably effective but should be tried (second generation non-sedating classes preferred).
- Phototherapy: Narrow-band UVB can help to decrease symptoms and skin involvement in some patients with eczema, perhaps via an immunosuppressive mechanism.
- Systemic immunosuppressives: For patients with severe or recalcitrant disease, systemic therapies such as methotrexate, mycophenolate mofetil, or cyclosporine can be helpful.

Integrative Treatment Options

- Environmental allergen reduction: Of equal importance in skin care management is providing a home environment that is allergen and irritant-free; as much as possible, carpets should be removed, curtains and furniture surfaces should be regularly cleared of dust, the presence of shedding pets should be reconsidered, and secondary smoke should be eliminated. It may also be helpful to place a cool-mist humidifier in patients' bedrooms, and attempt to avoid direct skin contact with wool and artificial textiles (prefer 100 % cotton).

- Acupuncture: Both acupuncture and acupressure have significant literature support as modalities to calm itching, perhaps via a direct anti-inflammatory mechanism [1, 2].
- Essential oils: Topical sunflower seed oil, with its high content of anti-inflammatory linoleic acid, and coconut oil, a good emollient with demonstrated antibacterial properties, have demonstrated utility in studies of atopic dermatitis [3–6].
- Hypnosis: Hypnosis exploits the mind-body connection and may have direct anti-inflammatory benefits, but also targets the stress response and may confer behavioral modifications to break the itch-scratch cycle [7].

Case Discussion The physician spent a great deal of time reviewing gentle skin care practices with the patient's mother, and provided a handout with recommend soap and emollient brands. It was also suggested that, perhaps in future visits, the patient's father could come to clinic appointments so that environmental issues in his home (such as the carpet and secondary smoke) could be addressed. The patient was given a prescription for tacrolimus 0.03 % ointment and mometasone 0.1 % ointment to use twice daily for 2 weeks on face and body (respectively), and was recommended to moisturize with coconut oil mixed with a ceramide-based cream (available over the counter). She was also given a 1-week course of systemic cephalexin in light of the impetiginized/crusted areas of skin, and was counseled to eat yogurt enriched with probiotics while on this therapy.

She was referred to a medical hypnotist, which her mother reported was the most effective method of reducing her desire to scratch. Subsequently, her skin healed and she was almost symptom-free at her 3 month follow-up.

References

1. Pfab F, Huss-Marp J, Gatti A, Fuqin J, Athanasiadis GI, Irnich D, et al. Influence of acupuncture on type I hypersensitivity itch and the wheal and flare response in adults with atopic eczema—a

blinded, randomized, placebo-controlled, crossover trial. Allergy. 2010;65:903–10.

2. Lee KC, Keyes A, Hensley JR, Gordon JR, Kwasny MJ, West DP, et al. Effectiveness of acupressure on pruritus and lichenification associated with atopic dermatitis: a pilot trial. Acupunct Med: J Br Med Acupunct Soc. 2012;30:8–11.

3. Agero AL, Verallo-Rowell VM. A randomized double-blind controlled trial comparing extra virgin coconut oil with mineral oil as a moisturizer for mild to moderate xerosis. Dermatitis. 2004;15(3):109–16.

4. Evangelista MT, Abad-Casintahan F, Lopez-Villafuerte L. The effect of topical virgin coconut oil on SCORAD index, transepidermal water loss, and skin capacitance in mild to moderate pediatric atopic dermatitis: a randomized, double-blind, clinical trial. Int J Dermatol. 2014;53(1):100–8.

5. Msika P, De Belilovsky C, Piccardi N, et al. New emollient with topical corticosteroid-sparing effect in treatment of childhood atopic dermatitis: SCORAD and quality of life improvement. Pediatr Dermatol. 2008;25(6):606–12.

6. Verallo-Rowell VM, Dillague KM, Syah-Tjundawan BS. Novel antibacterial and emollient effects of coconut and virgin olive oils in adult atopic dermatitis. Dermatitis. 2008;19(6):308–15.

7. Stewart AC, Thomas SE. Hypnotherapy as a treatment for atopic dermatitis in adults and children. Br J Dermatol. 1995;132: 778–83.

Chapter 11
64 Year Old Man Presents to the Office Asking for Evaluation of Lesions on His Ankles

Robert A. Norman, Patrick Brennan and Laura Jordan

Case Presentation

64 y/o man presents to the office asking for evaluation of lesions on his ankles. Patient complains of a heaviness in his legs that is worsened when standing still and at the end of the day. The patient explains that the lesion began this past winter, about 8 months ago, when his legs became dry, scaly, and pruritic. After the patient scratched the area, the lesion grew in size and became more irritated. Upon visual inspections, the patient's legs appear edematous and erythematous, and crusted scaly erosions are present bilaterally around his ankles. The patient has not had any prior treatment for the lesions. His past medical history is

R.A. Norman (✉)
Dermatology Healthcare, Tampa, FL, USA
e-mail: SkinDrRob@aol.com

P. Brennan • L. Jordan
Lake Erie College of Osteopathic Medicine,
Bradenton, FL, USA

R.A. Norman, R. Rupani, *Clinical Cases in Integrative Dermatology*, Clinical Cases in Dermatology 4, DOI 10.1007/978-3-319-10244-3_11, © Springer International Publishing Switzerland 2015

significant for varicose veins. He is not currently on any medications.

Differential Diagnosis

1. Stasis dermatitis
2. Asteatotic eczema
3. Atopic dermatitis
4. Cellulitis
5. Tinea pedis

Diagnosis   Stasis Dermatitis

Discussion

Overview of Stasis Dermatitis

Stasis Dermatitis stems from chronic venous insufficiency. Chronic edema and venous incompetence set the stage for the development of stasis dermatitis. Patients often exhibit a history of varicose veins and deep venous thrombosis. Other associated factors are pregnancy, increased blood volume, and increased venocaval pressure. Patients will classically first notice stasis dermatitis in the lower extremities over the medial ankles. The initial presenting symptoms here are erythema and pruritus.

During and acute inflammation stasis dermatitis can mimic cellulitis with evidence of exudate and crusting skin. In the chronic state, stasis dermatitis is known for exhibiting dermal fibrosis. The repetitive exudative extravasation of erythrocytes seen in chronic stasis dermatitis leads to progressive pigmentation of the skin from the hemosiderin deposits (Fig. 11.1). Complications of stasis dermatitis often include secondary infection as well as the maturation of venous stasis ulcers [1, 2].

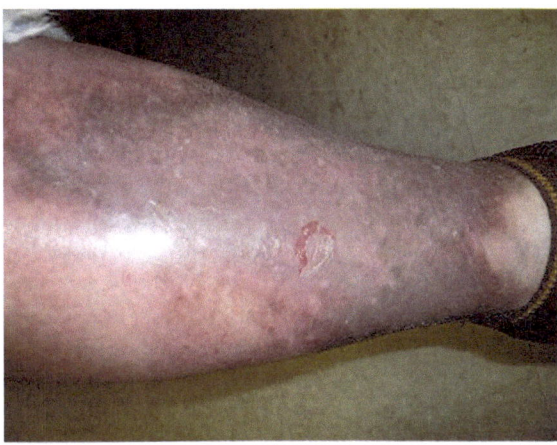

FIGURE 11.1 Severe stasis

Pathogenesis

The chronic venous insufficiency that leads to stasis dermatitis exhibits irregular venous flow patterns. Normally, valves of the deep veins in the calves block the retrograde flow of venous blood. Previous deep vein thrombosis can lead to post-thrombotic syndrome and incompetent valves of the deep veins of the lower extremities. Communicating veins that unite the superficial calf veins with the deep veins are also damaged in the setting of chronic venous insufficiency. In this case blood will demonstrate retrograde venous flow from the deep calf veins to the superficial venous plexuses. These irregular flow patterns contribute to the pathogenesis of stasis dermatitis.

Fibrin deposited in the face of this vascular damage also contributes to the disease process. Fibrin is laid down in the extravascular space causing sclerosis. The microvasculature and lymphatic channels become destroyed and nutrition of the epidermis is compromised. Eventually the epidermis breaks down and venous stasis ulcers arise [1, 2].

Clinical Presentation

Patients with stasis dermatitis often present with classic clinical signs of chronic venous insufficiency. As with our patient, they will often complain of aches, pains, and heaviness of the legs. These symptoms are provoked by periods of standing still and are relieved by walking. The use of leg musculature helps pump the blood through these compromised vasculature structures. Edema of the legs is also associated with standing and is worst at the end of the day. Patients' shoes fit tightly by the end of the day as a result of the edema and they often experience night cramps. The edema often resolves or improves to some degree in the morning after the patient has experienced an extended period of time in a horizontal position while sleeping. This position takes the pressure off of the veins with nonfunctional valves [1, 2].

Crusted and scaly erosions are often seen around the ankles. Inflammatory papules may be present. Dermal sclerosis may also be present and can be painful and limit movement of the ankle. Varying degrees of pigmentation is also noticeable due to hemosiderin deposits from old and new hemorrhages. Pruritus associated with stasis dermatitis may lead to excoriations from chronic scratching. Irritant dermatitis may also be simultaneously present as a result of secretions from venous stasis ulcers and bacterial colonization [1, 2].

Venous stasis ulcers are a frequent complication of chronic venous stasis and stasis dermatitis. These ulcers are frequently found on the calf. Most commonly near the medial malleolus. They are described as irregularly shaped with well-defined boarders. They are usually shallow but can be quite large and possibly involve the entire circumference of the lower leg. Venous stasis ulcers are painful and are usually roofed with necrotic tissue. There is virtually always secondary bacterial colonization and rarely squamous cell carcinoma can develop from a chronic ulcer [2, 3].

Laboratory Examinations and Diagnosis

The diagnosis of stasis dermatitis can usually be made with a thorough history and clinical examination. Doppler, color-coded duplex sonography, and venography can also aid in diagnosis.

Venography is a study the uses X-ray to locate thrombi in the venous system. It is performed by injecting dye into the venous system of the examined extremity and then taking X-ray films at timed intervals. Absence of the dye from progressing through the venous system indicates an occlusion. In this way, the venous system is visualized for patency. Venography is accurate for diagnosing thrombi below the knee [4].

Doppler ultrasound is useful for detecting the movement of red blood cells within veins. It is able to detect venous occlusion. The characteristic swish sound of the patent venous system is absent in the face of venous occlusion. However, the Doppler ultrasound does not provide accurate results for occlusion below the upper calf. A color-coded duplex sonogram allows for a pulsed Doppler probe within the transducer to assess both blood flow velocity and direction. A color is allocated for direction of blood flow within the vessel. The intensity of the color is related to the velocity of the blood traveling in the vessel. Thus, slowing of blood or reversal of its direction can be visualized and venous insufficiency can be detected [4].

Treatment

Stasis dermatitis can be greatly improved by the simple treatment of leg elevation routinely throughout the course of the day. The use of compression stockings is also beneficial. The stockings should have a minimal gradient of 30 mmHg in order to be effective. Midpotency topical steroids and emollients are also useful. Patients should be instructed to protect the areas from injury and avoid scratching. The edema may need diuretics for control.

Venous ulcers can be problematic to treat once they occur. All necrotic tissue that develops over the ulcer should be carefully debrided periodically and covered with a semipermeable compression dressing. Steroids will prolong the healing process of venous ulcers and should not be applied in these areas. Oral and topical antibiotic therapy should be instituted if the area becomes secondarily infected. Pentoxifylline may be added to treat the symptoms of intermittent claudication resulting from peripheral artery disease [5]. Skin grafts may be necessary in the face of chronic ulcers [1, 2].

Integrative Approach

Herbal remedies for stasis dermatitis exist. Prepared forms of the deciduous horse-chestnut tree are used by some herbalists to treat venous insufficiency. Proanthocyanidins, tannins, and saponins are the active ingredients that work to constrict veins and improve the venous circulatory problems seen in stasis dermatitis [6].

Aloe vera is a plant of Africa that contains leaves full of salve. This ointment contains enzymes that have anti-inflammatory properties that promote wound healing. Topical application of the aloe vera salve may help heal the venous ulcers associated with stasis dermatitis and also relieve some of the pruritus associated with the condition [7].

Calendula is an herb that has a history of usefulness in treating ulcers. It is used by herbalists for its anti-inflammatory and would healing properties. Calendula is used in stasis dermatitis to reduce the risk of infection and to promote the growth of granulation tissue in ulcers to speed the healing process [6].

References

1. Fauci AS, et al. Harrison's principles of internal medicine. 17th ed. New York: McGraw-Hill; 2008. p. 314–16. 335, 366, 731.
2. Wolff K, Johnson RA. Fitzpatrick's color atlas & synopsis of clinical dermatology. 6th ed. New York: McGraw-Hill Companies; 2009. p. 465–77.
3. Gyton AC, Hall JE. Textbook of medical physiology. 11th ed. Philadelphia: Elsevier; 2006. p. 459–67.
4. Pagana KD, Pagana TJ. Mosby's manual of diagnostic and laboratory tests. 3rd ed. St. Louis: Mosby Elsevier; 2006. p. 949–52. 1163–5.
5. Salhiyyah K, Senanayake E, Abdel-Hadi M, Booth A, Michaels JA. Pentoxifylline for intermittent claudication. Cochrane Database Syst Rev 1(1): CD005262.
6. Wink M, van Wyk B-E. Medicinal plants of the world. New York: Timber Press; 2004.
7. Balch JF, Balch PA. Prescription for nutritional healing. 5th ed. Philadelphia: Penguin; 2010.

Chapter 12
A 35-Year-Old Woman Presented to the Office Asking for Evaluation of Lesions on the Back of Her Neck and Lower Legs

Robert A. Norman and Laura Jordan

Case Presentation

A 35-year-old woman presented to the office asking for evaluation of lesions on the back of her neck and lower legs. The patient complained of pruritus at the lesion site and stated that the lesions began as small and red, but after about a month they grew together and darkened. She complained that she could not stop scratching the areas and believed she could have been scratching in her sleep. She has had these lesions now for 4 months and affirms that they have not grown in size. Upon physical exam, the lesions appeared dark and lichenified with superficial bright red excoriations.

R.A. Norman (✉)
Dermatology Healthcare, Tampa, FL, USA
e-mail: SkinDrRob@aol.com

L. Jordan
Lake Erie College of Osteopathic Medicine,
Bradenton, FL, USA

R.A. Norman, R. Rupani, *Clinical Cases in Integrative Dermatology*, Clinical Cases in Dermatology 4, DOI 10.1007/978-3-319-10244-3_12,
© Springer International Publishing Switzerland 2015

The patient had attempted OTC corticosteroid cream with minimal improvement. She is not on any other medications, and her past medical history is remarkable for generalized anxiety disorder. The patient also mentioned that she was currently going through a difficult divorce.

Differential Diagnosis

1. Neurodermatitis
2. Asteatotic eczema
3. Psoriasis

Asteatotic eczema occurs most commonly on the lower legs and appears as dry and scaly with xerosis, and over time red plaques emerge with thin, long horizontal superficial fissures. Although this patient has lesions on her lower legs, she also has lesions on the nape of her neck, an uncommon area in asteatotic eczema. Psoriasis also can present with pruritus of the lower legs; however, this patient does not present with the classic psoriatic thick, silvery scaled lesions.

Diagnosis   Neurodermatitis

Discussion

Overview

Neurodermatitis, also known as lichen simplex chronicus, is a condition in which habitual scratching of a localized area creates an eczematous eruption. The lesions remain localized and do not tend to enlarge. Over time, red papules coalesce and lichenify. The most common sites for neurodermatitis are areas which are easily reached like the nape of the neck, the lower legs and ankles, the sides of the neck, the scalp, the upper thighs, the vulva, pubis or scrotum, and the extensor forearms (Fig. 12.1).

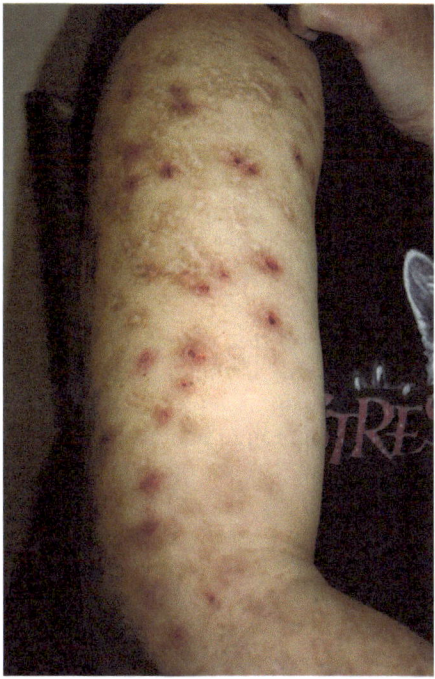

FIGURE 12.1 Neurodermatitis

This disorder is common in people with skin allergies, eczema, psoriasis, or psychological issues like anxiety and depression. Women are more likely to develop neurodermatitis, and the onset is most common between 30 and 50 years of age. It is also common among children who are unable to stop scratching an insect bite or who have other pruritic skin disorders [1–3].

A primary concern for these lesions is risk of infection and permanent scarring, so they should be monitored on a continual basis. Additionally, a study has shown that patients with neurodermatitis may also suffer from other comorbidities such as sexual dysfunction and depression [1, 2, 4].

Pathogenesis

Patients with neurodermatitis experience a vicious cycle. Their lesions may start with a small irritation to the area, and the patient begins to scratch the itchy area. This constant scratching causes the skin to thicken, and this thickened skin itches which causes more scratching and greater thickening. In this way, patients find relief from scratching the inflamed site and continued subconscious scratching may lead to the recurring eruption [1, 2, 5].

Solak et al. also found that damage to the peripheral nervous system played a role in the etiology of neurodermatitis on the limbs, finding that nerve root compression and radiculopathy were more common in patients with neurodermatitis. As such, these patients should be examined for a possible underlying neuropathy [3].

Clinical Presentation

A patient normally presents with chronic itching of the skin which increases in times of stress. The skin may appear as a lichenified, dark patch or plaque commonly located in easy to reach areas of the body. The skin may also appear raw with fresh scratch marks and scaling [1, 5].

Laboratory Examinations and Diagnosis

The diagnosis of neurodermatitis is based on a patient's history of itching and scratching and examination of their skin. A physician may biopsy the affected site to rule out other pruritic conditions [2].

Treatment

The primary goal of treatment is to break the itch-scratch cycle. Physicians may prescribe corticosteroids (Clobetasol) or anti-histamines to relieve the pruritus. Additionally, nodules caused by picking at the scalp may require intralesional injections with triamcinolone acetonide.

Anti-anxiety drugs may also aid in a patient's recovery as anxiety and stress are usually triggers for this disorder. If a patient acquires a bacterial infection at the affected site, the physician may prescribe antibiotics. Finally, patients may also benefit from treatment of any underlying psychiatric conditions by seeking the care of a mental health professional [1, 2].

Integrative Approach

Many home remedies exist to help neurodermatitis patients break their scratching habit. For example, covering the affected area with bandages can place a barrier between the affected area and their scratching hand, an especially important maneuver if the patient is a subconscious night scratcher. Patients may also choose to keep their nails short in order to minimize the damage to their skin. Taking cool baths and adding in baking soda or oatmeal may sooth the skin, and wearing smooth-textured cotton clothing can avoid irritating the skin. Patients should try to choose mild soaps without dyes or perfumes as well as keep their stress under control as stress is often a trigger for this disorder [2]. Guided meditation, relaxation and breathing techniques (see previous chapters), and self-hypnosis are excellent to aid in improvement. Camphor is derived from a distillate of the wood of the Camphor tree (*Cinnamomum camphora*) and is an effective antipruritic. Menthol is derived from Japanese mint *(Mentha arvensis)* and has a cooling antipruritic and antibacterial effect. Oats (*Avena sativa*) have been used in baths for hundreds of years for their soothing and antipruritic properties. Aloe vera is effective to decrease inflammation and promote healing. Saint John's wort (Hypericum perforatum) can improve mild to moderate depression but significantly interacts with the metabolism of a number of other drugs. Valerian (Valariana spp.) is helpful for insomnia and anxiety.

Additionally, Engin et al. found that transcutaneous electrical nerve stimulation (TENS) may also offer an alternative treatment for neurodermatitis by decreasing pruritis in patients [6].

Key Points

1. Neurodermatitis, also known as lichen simplex chronicus, is a condition in which habitual scratching of a localized area creates an eczematous eruption.
2. The most common sites for neurodermatitis are areas which are easily reached.
3. Women are more likely to develop neurodermatitis, and the onset is most common between 30 and 50 years of age.
4. Patients may benefit from dermatological, psychiatric, and integrative therapy to treat this disorder.

References

1. Habif TP. Clinical dermatology: a color guide to diagnosis and therapy. 5th ed. Hanover: Elsevier; 2010.
2. Harms RW. Psoriasis: alternative medicine. In: Bauer BA, Gibson LE, editors. MayoClinic. 2012. Retrieved on 4 Sept 2013 from http://www.mayoclinic.com/health/psoriasis/DS00193/DSECTION=alternative-medicine
3. Solak O, Kulac M, Yaman M, Karaca S, Toktas H, Kirpiko O, Kavuncu V. Lichen simplex chronicus as a symptom of neuropathy. Clin Exp Dermatol. 2009;34(4):476–80. doi:10.1111/j.1365-2230.2008.02969.x.
4. Mercan S, Altunay I, Demir B, Akpinar A, Kayaoglu S. Sexual dysfunctions in patients with neurodermatitis and psoriasis. J Sex Marital Ther. 2008;34(2):160–8. doi:10.1080/00926230701267951.
5. Berman K. Lichen simplex chronicus. MedlinePlus. 2012. Retrieved on 4 Sept 2013 from http://www.nlm.nih.gov/medlineplus/ency/article/000872.htm
6. Engin B, Tufekci O, Yazici A, Ozdemir M. The effect of transcutaneous electrical nerve stimulation in the treatment of lichen simplex: a prospective study. Clin Exp Dermatol. 2009;34(3):324–8. doi:10.1111/j.1365-2230.2008.03086.x.

Chapter 13
A 66-Year-Old Man Presented to the Office Asking for Evaluation of a Lesion on His Nose

Robert A. Norman and Laura Jordan

Case Presentation

A 66-year-old man presented to the office asking for evaluation of a lesion on his nose. The patient explained that the lesion had been present for over a year, had a history of bleeding and then scabbing over, and had grown slightly in size. Upon visual inspection, the lesion appeared as a smooth pearly pink papule with telangiectatic vessels. The patient had not had any prior treatment for the lesion. His past medical history was significant for sunburns as a child as well as extensive sun exposure as a retired construction worker.

R.A. Norman (✉)
Dermatology Healthcare, Tampa, FL, USA
e-mail: SkinDrRob@aol.com

L. Jordan
Lake Erie College of Osteopathic Medicine,
Bradenton, FL, USA

R.A. Norman, R. Rupani, *Clinical Cases in Integrative Dermatology*, Clinical Cases in Dermatology 4, DOI 10.1007/978-3-319-10244-3_13, © Springer International Publishing Switzerland 2015

Differential Diagnosis

1. Nodular basal cell carcinoma
2. Actinic keratosis
3. Fibrous papule
4. Molluscum contagiosum

Diagnosis   Nodular basal cell carcinoma

Actinic keratosis can serve as precursors to squamous cell carcinomas, appearing as flat, pink lesions that feel like sandpaper. This patient's lesion is raised and smooth with visible vessels. A fibrous papule is a benign lesion which usually develops late in adolescence or early adult life on the nose. It can be differentiated from a basal cell carcinoma because it does not have a tendency to grow in size, bleed, or ulcerate. Molluscum contagiosum is a viral infection of the skin that usually occurs in children and presents as round, firm, painless bumps. Unlike this lesion, molluscum tends to occur in groups and usually clears in 12–18 months without treatment. Ultimately, the definitive diagnosis for this patient's lesion will be histological analysis of a biopsy sample.

Discussion

Overview

Two major types of nonmelanocytic skin tumors exist: basal cell carcinoma (BCC) and squamous cell carcinoma (SCC).

BCCs have a lower tendency to metastasize than SCCs. Nevertheless, if left untreated, they can advance by direct extension and destroy the entire side of the face or invade tissue into the bone and brain. Both BCCs and SCCs are more common in men than women, and caucasians have a 30 % lifetime risk of developing a BCC and a 9–14 % (men) or 4–9 % (women) lifetime risk of developing a SCC. Patients with a history of BCC are at a higher risk of developing more lesions with approximately 40 % developing a subsequent lesion in less than 5 years.

Risk factors for developing both BCCs and SCCs include living close to the equator, UV light exposure, indoor tanning, history of sunburns, and having fair skin and light eyes. Although UV light exposure is the most important cause of BCC, one third of BCCs emerge in areas that are protected from the sun. For SCCs, immunocompromised patients are at greater risk. For example, renal transplant patients have a 253-fold higher risk of SCC [1–4].

Pathogenesis

BCC develops from basal keratinocytes of the epidermis after DNA has been damaged by UVB radiation. They require surrounding stroma for their growth by direct extension and are not able to metastasize through blood or lymphatics. BCCs are unpredictable in that they may remain small for years or grow rapidly. BCCs have also been linked to the PTCH1 gene mutation in patients with familial basal cell nevus syndrome, xeroderma pigmentosum, as well as sporadic disease which requires two gene mutations.

SCCs develop from keratinocytes in the epidermis, creating a lesion which can infiltrate the dermis. They have the ability to spread via expansion, shelving, conduit spread, or metastasis. Metastasis begins mainly via regional lymph node spread, but distant spread may continue via hematogenous dissemination. Potential for metastasis is increased with size greater than 2 cm, depth greater than 4 mm, poor differentiation, location on the ear or lip, previous treatment, perineural involvement, and immunosuppression [1, 3, 4].

Clinical Presentation

BCCs are the most common malignancy in Caucasians (they are uncommon in blacks) and the most common invasive malignant cutaneous cancer in humans. Generally, they present as a recurring bleeding or scabbing sore on the head and neck region with the nose serving as the most common site. BCCs may also appear in sites protected from the sun like the genitals and breasts.

BCCs occur in a variety of clinical presentations.

Nodular BCC is the most common type and presents as a pearly pink papule with telangiectatic vessels. A history of the lesion ulcerating and then healing is common. A variant of nodular BCC is cystic BCC.

Pigmented BCCs must have at least one of the following features: large gray-blue ovoid nests, multiple gray-blue globules, maple leaf-like areas, spoke wheel areas, ulceration, and "treelike" telangiectasia.

Sclerosing or morpheaform BCC which appears waxy, firm, possibly slightly raised, and pale white or yellow in color.

Superficial BCC is slow-growing and occurs mostly on the trunk and extremities and appears as an oval, red, scaling plaque with raised pearly white borders.

SCCs are the second most common cancer among Caucasians. They also appear in sun-exposed areas and are more common on the scalp, backs of the hands, and the ear. The most common precursor lesion to SCCs is actinic keratosis, which begins as a rough, flat, pink lesion which feels like sandpaper. SCCs which arise from actinic keratosis can be freely moveable with a thick, adherent scale and an erythematous base. Those which do not arise from actinic keratosis have little surface scale. Bowen's disease is another form of SCC which presents as red, smooth plaques on the glans penis [1, 3, 4].

Laboratory Examinations and Diagnosis

Diagnosis for BCC and SCC can be made upon clinical examination, followed by histological confirmation via skin biopsy.

Treatment

Treatment options for BCC and SCC include electrodesiccation and curettage (ED&C), excision surgery, Mohs surgery, focal radiation therapy, or topical imiquimod or 5-fluorouracil creams.

ED&C is preferred for BCCs on the trunk and extremities which do not have high-risk features and for SCCs evolving from actinic keratosis. This treatment involves a cycle of electrodesiccation followed by curettage usually repeated one to three times until normal tissue can be distinguished by the curette. A hypopigmented scar may result.

Excision surgery is preferred for BCCs with definitive borders on the trunk, legs, cheeks, and forehead and for SCCs which are larger or near the vermilion border of the lips. Cosmetic result is better than ED&C, and healing time is faster.

Mohs surgery is a microscopically controlled technique that is preferred for sclerosing BCCs, BCCs without defined margins, and SCCs that penetrate through the dermis. When SCCs metastasize, treatment should combine Mohs surgery with sentinel lymphadenectomy.

Radiation therapy is useful in patients who are unable to tolerate surgical procedures.

Topical imiquimod 5 % modifies the immune response and can be used 5–7 times per week for 6 weeks to treat superficial BCC or daily application for 6–16 weeks to treat Bowen's disease. 5-fluorouracil can be used 2 times daily for up to 12 weeks to treat superficial BCCs or 2 times daily for 2–3 weeks for actinic keratosis [1, 4, 5].

Integrative Approach

Alternative therapies may be used toward preventing skin cancer. Patients can increase their vitamin D levels and modify their diet to include fresh, raw, unprocessed foods containing beta-carotene (spinach, kale), lycopene (tomatoes), lutein (spinach, kale), epigallocatechin gallate and polyphenols (green and black tea), flavonoids (citrus), proanthocyanadins (cocoa), and cruciferous vegetables. Additionally, antioxidants (including vitamin C, vitamin E, beta-carotene, zinc, and vitamin A), folic acid, and selenium may help prevent the development of skin cancer. Herbs have also been identified as preventative therapy like camellia sinensis from green tea which contains polyphenols, bilberry, ginkgo, milk thistle, ginger and hawthorn.

In addition to preventative therapy, some alternative therapies have been argued to treat already present skin cancer. For example, extract from the plants of Solanaceae family (which include eggplant, tomato, potato), known as solasodine rhamnosyl glycosides (BEC) or BEC5, has been argued to cure most non-melanocytic skin cancers in several weeks [6, 7].

Key Points

1. Basal cell carcinoma and squamous cell carcinoma are two major types of nonmelanocytic skin tumors with basal cell serving as the most common.
2. Squamous cell carcinoma has a greater risk of metastasis and a stronger relationship to UVB radiation than basal cell carcinoma.
3. Treatment of both cancers include electrodesiccation and curettage (ED&C), excision surgery, Mohs surgery, focal radiation therapy, or topical imiquimod or 5-fluorouracil creams.
4. Preventative alternative therapies exist for both cancers including diet, supplements, and herbs.
5. Eggplant extract has been argued to treat non-melanocytic skin cancers.

References

1. Habif TP. Clinical dermatology: a color guide to diagnosis and therapy. 5th ed. Hanover: Elsevier; 2010.

2. Harms RW. Skin cancer. In: Bauer BA, Gibson LE, editors. MayoClinic. 2012. Retrieved on 14 Sept 2013 from http://www.mayoclinic.com/health/skin-cancer/DS00190

3. Lim JL, Asgari M. Clinical features and diagnosis of cutaneous squamous cell carcinoma. UpToDate. 2013. Retrieved on 15 Sept 2013 from http://www.uptodate.com.lecomlrc.lecom.edu/contents/clinical-features-and-diagnosis-of-cutaneous-squamous-cell-carcinoma-scc?detectedLanguage=en&source=search_resul t&search=squamous+cell+carcinoma&selectedTitle=1~150&pro vider=noProvider

4. Wu PA. Epidemiology and clinical features of basal cell carcinoma. UpToDate. 2013. Retrieved on 15 Sept 2013 from http://www.uptodate.com.lecomlrc.lecom.edu/contents/epidemiology-and-clinical-features-of-basal-cell-carcinoma?detectedLanguage =en&source=search_result&search=basal+cell+carcinoma&sele ctedTitle=1~128&provider=noProvider

5. Jorizzo J. Treatment of actinic keratosis. UpToDate. 2013. Retrieved on 15 Sept 2013 from http://www.uptodate.com.lecomlrc.lecom. edu/contents/treatment-of-actinic-keratosis?source=see_ link&anchor=H11#H11

6. Ehrlich SD. Skin cancer. University of Maryland Medical Center. 2012. Retrieved on 15 Sept 2013 from http://umm.edu/health/medical/altmed/condition/skin-cancer

7. Mercola J. BEC or eggplant extract: stunning new way to flush away skin cancer. 2011. Retrieved on 15 Sept 2013 from http://articles.mercola.com/sites/articles/archive/2011/12/10/vitamin-d-exposure-possible-natural-cure-for-skin-cancers.aspx

Chapter 14
A 22-Year-Old Hispanic Woman Presented to the Office Asking for Evaluation of a Rash on Her Face

Robert A. Norman and Laura Jordan

Case Presentation

A 22-year-old Hispanic woman presented to the office asking for evaluation of a rash on her face. The patient complained that the rash appeared on her nose and cheeks after brief sun exposure and lasted for nearly a week. She stated that this has occurred on multiple occasions within this past year. Physical exam revealed a superficial erythematous plaque on the nasal bridge and cheekbones. The patient admitted that she was not diligent about applying sunscreen on her face in the past. She is not on any medications, and her family history is remarkable for rheumatoid arthritis in her mother and lupus in her maternal grandmother.

R.A. Norman (✉)
Dermatology Healthcare, Tampa, FL, USA
e-mail: SkinDrRob@aol.com

L. Jordan
Lake Erie College of Osteopathic Medicine,
Bradenton, FL, USA

R.A. Norman, R. Rupani, *Clinical Cases in Integrative*   107
Dermatology, Clinical Cases in Dermatology 4,
DOI 10.1007/978-3-319-10244-3_14,
© Springer International Publishing Switzerland 2015

Differential Diagnosis

1. Dermatomyositis
2. Cutaneous lupus erythematosus
3. Rosacea
4. Seborrheic dermatitis

Diagnosis Cutaneous lupus erythematosus

Discussion

Dermatomyositis is an inflammatory disease of the skin and skeletal muscles. Although the muscular inflammation can occur after the cutaneous manifestations in this disease, the patient did not present with the characteristic skin involvement of the hands and knuckles of dermatomyositis, making this diagnosis less likely. Rosacea often occurs after the age of 30 and often appears with papules and pustules. Although this patient's lesion was located in an area common for rosacea, the diagnosis is less likely. Finally, seborrheic dermatitis can present as a red lesion over the malar region of the face; however, it may also present with dry, yellow scale at the inflamed base which this patient did not have.

Overview

Systemic lupus erythematosus (SLE) is a multisystem connective tissue disease affecting the blood, joints, skin, and kidneys. It primarily affects women in their 20s and 30s with a higher incidence in blacks and Hispanics. The severity of this disease is highly variable and may present with exacerbations and remissions throughout a patient's life. Common symptoms include fatigue, fever, and arthralgia, and approximately 50 %

of patients present with cutaneous features including a butterfly rash, discoid lupus, and photosensitivity [1–3].

Pathogenesis

The onset of SLE has been linked to genetics and the environment. Greater risk of developing SLE exists for patients whose family members have the disease. Environmental factors which exacerbate SLE or precipitate its onset include UV light exposure, infections, estrogen, medications, stress, surgery, and pregnancy. Such factors may lead to cell destruction and creation of antibodies against nuclear antigens. Further, an allele of STAT4, a transcription factor used in mediating responses to IL-12 in lymphocytes and in regulation of T helper cell differentiation, is associated with increased risk for SLE [1–3].

Clinical Presentation

Cutaneous lupus erythematosus can more commonly present as a rash, telangiectasia, alopecia, utricaria, or Raynaud's phenomenon.

Cutaneous lupus erythematosus rash can be subdivided into several subsets: discoid lupus erythematosus (DLE) in 25 % of patients, subacute cutaneous LE (SCLE) in 10 % of patients, and acute cutaneous LE in 50 % of patients. Chronic discoid lesions can occur in up to 25 % of lupus patients, and patients with these lesions have a 5–10 % greater risk of developing systemic symptoms of lupus. These lesions appear well-formed red plaques which are covered with scale that infiltrates the hair follicles. These lesions most frequently occur on sun-exposed areas. SCLE lesions start out as small red papules with slight scaling that become either psoriasiform or ringed form. The acute cutaneous lupus erythematosus rash is the classic malar rash on the cheeks and nose which occurs normally after UV light exposure.

Telangiectasias occur in 53 % of lupus patients and present on the palms and fingers but spare the knuckles. Alopecia occurs in more than 20 % of lupus patients and can be scarring or nonscarring, with the latter being more common in lupus. Utricaria occurs between 7 and 28 % in lupus patients and my not be visually distinct from hives; however, the urticarial lesions in lupus are non-pruritic and stay in the same location as opposed to hives. Lastly, Raynaud's phenomenon occurs in greater than 20 % of lupus patients and can appear before other signs of the disease by months to years.

In neonatal lupus erythematosis, infants develop red macules, patches, or plaques soon after birth which are worsened by UV light exposure. This syndrome is rare and is associated with maternal antibodies to Ro/SSA, La/SSB, or U1RNP and usually resolves within 6–8 months [2, 4].

Laboratory Examinations and Diagnosis

Patients with cutaneous LE should have their lesion biopsied in order to define the type of cutaneous lesion. Additionally, patients can have a biopsy performed on their normal (lesion free) sun-exposed skin to have a Lupus band test performed. For patients with DLE, SCLE, or SLE, immunoglobulin deposits will be located at the dermoepidermal junction. Further, such patients should obtain blood studies to evaluate their disease progression over time. Patients with cutaneous manifestations of lupus should be evaluated for manifestations of SLE such as renal, hematologic, neurologic, or immunologic disorders because they have a higher risk of developing SLE. Such studies include: CBC, ESR, platelet count, ANA, anti-nDNA, anti-RNP, anti-Ro, anti-La, anti-Smith, serologic tests, and urinalysis. To be diagnosed with SLE, they would need to have 4 of the following 11 parameters: malar rash, discoid rash, photosensitivity, oral ulcers, arthritis, serositis, renal disorder, neurologic disorder, hematologic disorder, immunologic disorder, and ANA [2, 5].

Treatment

Preventative care for patients with cutaneous LE includes avoidance of direct exposure to sunlight and sunscreen with a value greater than 15 SPF. Topical corticosteroids are the first line agents for cutaneous LE. Patients may apply corticosteroids up to three times a day, limiting it to the affected area. DLE lesions may be resistant to topical steroids. Topical tacrolimus has been shown to be effective. Certain recalcitrant lesions may respond better to intralesional steroid injections [6].

When topical steroids fail, antimalarial agents are the drugs of choice to treat cutaneous LE. Patients can be maintained on a therapeutic dosage of hydroxychloroquine two times a day until their lesions resolve, after which they should be reduced to the lowest dosage and maintained to moderate flare-ups. An important concern which accompanies the use of antimalarial agents is ocular, specifically retinal, toxicity. Thus, patients should have periodic eye exams. Dapsone is an alternative to antimalarials to treat cutaneous LE.

When patients fail to respond to topical steroids, antimalarial agents, or dapsone, they may switch to oral corticosteroids. Patients are put on high dose prednisone until their disease is controlled and then slowly tapered and moved back to traditional therapy.

Other alternative drug therapies include azathioprine, methotrexate, thalidomide, and acitretin for resistant DLE; isoretinoin for DLE and SCLE; and mycophenolate mofetil for refractory dermatologic conditions of SLE [2, 4, 5].

Integrative Approach

Patients with cutaneous LE may explore alternative treatments for their condition such as inclusion of herbs, dietary investigation and changes, and pulsed dye laser therapy.

Patients may include anti-inflammatory herbs in their diet to reduce their inflammation such as pine bark extract, grapeseed extract, turmeric, and reishi mushroom extract. They should avoid the herb Echinacea because it stimulates their immune system and would worsen their autoimmune disease.

Patients should strive to eat a low-calorie, low-fat diet, with less beef and dairy products and more vegetables, chicken, and especially fish. They should also drink eight glasses of water daily and research any food sensitivities which may be worsening their disease. Patients should avoid eating alfalfa, as this food stimulates the immune system with its compound L-canavanine, and plants in the nightshade family. Finally, patients should remove animal fats and oils high in omega-6 which also can increase inflammation [7].

Patients with refractory chronic DLE can try pulsed dye laser therapy (PDL). In Erceg et al.'s study, 12 patients with DLE received PDL therapy 3 times with a 6 week interval and 6 week follow-up period. The study found that PDL treatment is beneficial and safe for this population [8].

Key Points

1. Systemic lupus erythematosus (SLE) is a multisystem connective tissue disease affecting the blood, joints, skin, and kidneys. It primarily affects women in their 20s and 30s with a higher incidence in blacks and Hispanics. The onset of SLE has been linked to genetics and the environment.
2. Cutaneous lupus erythematosus can more commonly present as a rash, telangiectasia, alopecia, utricaria, or Raynaud's phenomenon.
3. Cutaneous lupus erythematosus rash can be subdivided into several subsets: discoid lupus erythematosus (DLE) in 25 % of patients, subacute cutaneous LE (SCLE) in 10 % of patients, and acute cutaneous LE in 50 % of patients.
4. Patients with cutaneous LE should have their lesion biopsied in order to define the type of cutaneous lesion. Additionally, patients can have a biopsy performed on their normal (lesion free) sun-exposed skin to have a Lupus band test performed.

5. Patients with cutaneous manifestations of lupus should be evaluated for manifestations of SLE such as renal, hematologic, neurologic, or immunologic disorders because they have a higher risk of developing SLE.
6. Preventative care for patients with cutaneous LE includes avoidance of direct exposure to sunlight and sunscreen with a value greater than 15 SPF.
7. Topical corticosteroids are the first line agents for cutaneous LE. When patients fail topical steroids they may move on to antimalarial agents or dapsone. If these agents fail, they may try oral corticosteroids.
8. Patients with cutaneous LE may explore alternative treatments for their condition such as inclusion of herbs, dietary investigation and changes, and pulsed dye laser therapy.

References

1. Goljan EF. Rapid review pathology. 3rd ed. Philadelphia: Elsevier; 2011.
2. Habif TP. Clinical dermatology: a color guide to diagnosis and therapy. 5th ed. Hanover: Elsevier; 2010.
3. Schur PH, Gladman DD. Overview of the clinical manifestations of systemic lupus erythematosus in adults. UpToDate. 2013. Retrieved on 17 Sept 2013 from http://www.uptodate.com. lecomlrc.lecom.edu/contents/overview-of-the-clinical-manifestations-of-systemic-lupus-erythematosus-in-adults?detec tedLanguage=en&source=search_result&search=lupus&selecte dTitle=1~150&provider=noProvider
4. Schur PH, Moschella SL. Mucocutaneous manifestations of systemic lupus erythematosis. UpToDate. 2013. Retrieved on 17 Sept 2013 from http://www.uptodate.com.lecomlrc.lecom.edu/con tents/mucocutaneous-manifestations-of-systemic-lupus-erythem atosus?detectedLanguage=en&source=search_result&search=c utaneous+lupus&selectedTitle=1~150&provider=noProvider
5. Lazaro D. Systemic lupus erythematosus. ACP smart medicine. 2013. Retrieved on 12 Oct 2013 from http://smartmedicine.acpon-line.org/content.aspx?gbosId=153&resultClick=3&ClientActionTy pe=SOLR%20Direct%20to%20Content&ClientActionData=syst

6. Heffernan MP, Nelson MM, Smith DI, Chung JH. 0.1% tacrolimus ointment in the treatment of discoid lupus erythematosus. Arch Dermatol. 2005;141(9):1170–1. doi:10.1001/archderm.141.9.1170.
7. Silverman C. Home remedies for lupus. The homemade medicine home remedies site. 2013. Retrieved on 12 Oct 2013 from http://www.homemademedicine.com/home-remedies-lupus.html
8. Erceg A, Bovenschen HJ, van de Kerkof PC, de Jong EM, Seyger MM. Efficacy and safety of pulsed dye laser treatment for cutaneous discoid lupus erythematosus. J Am Acad Dermatol. 2009;60(4):626–32. doi:10.1016/j.jaad.2008.11.904.

Index